The Power to Change Everything

THE
POWER
TO
CHANGE
EVERYTHING

The Small, Everyday Lifestyle
Changes That Will Help You
Crush Enormous Goals

CASEY ELKINS

NEW YORK

LONDON • NASHVILLE • MELBOURNE • VANCOUVER

The Power to Change Everything

The Small, Everyday Lifestyle Changes That Will Help You Crush Enormous Goals

Published in New York, New York, by Morgan James Publishing. Morgan James is a trademark of Morgan James, LLC. www.MorganJamesPublishing.com

Proudly distributed by Publishers Group West®

Scripture quotations are from the NIV Bible (The Holy Bible, New International Version), © 1979 Biblica, a nonprofit ministry and Zondervan Publishing. Used by permission. All rights reserved.

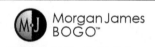

Morgan James BOGO™

A **FREE** ebook edition is available for you or a friend with the purchase of this print book.

CLEARLY SIGN YOUR NAME ABOVE

Instructions to claim your free ebook edition:
1. Visit MorganJamesBOGO.com
2. Sign your name CLEARLY in the space above
3. Complete the form and submit a photo of this entire page
4. You or your friend can download the ebook to your preferred device

ISBN 9781636982441 paperback
ISBN 9781636982458 ebook
Library of Congress Control Number: 2023939167

Cover & Interior Design by:
Christopher Kirk
www.GFSstudio.com

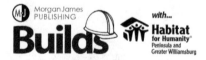

Morgan James is a proud partner of Habitat for Humanity Peninsula and Greater Williamsburg. Partners in building since 2006.

Get involved today! Visit: www.morgan-james-publishing.com/giving-back

To Brittany

Thank you for being my constant supporter, cheerleader, and voice of reason. I wouldn't be a portion of the man I am today without you by my side.

TABLE OF CONTENTS

FOREWORD

I t is my great honor to write the foreword for this inspiring book about Casey Elkins' journey to achieve the unimaginable. Overcoming numerous health obstacles, Casey achieved a feat many would consider impossible—completing multiple Ironman events.

For the uninformed, I thought it would be beneficial to know exactly what an Ironman is. The Ironman race is not for the faint of heart, as it requires a significant amount of training and preparation. Participants must be able to swim 2.4 miles, bike 112 miles, and run a full marathon (26.2 miles) *in a single day*, making it a physically and mentally demanding challenge. Just for context, I don't like to drive my car 112 miles, much less ride a bike… just before I run 26 miles. Can I get an "Amen"?

Given the rigorous nature of the event, the probability of participating in an Ironman is relatively low, unless you are well-prepared and have the necessary physical and mental fortitude to complete one. Casey signed up for his first Ironman when he was 100 pounds overweight. This is a small snippet for what's to come in the book. Spoiler alert: Casey went on to compete in 17-Ironman triathlons over a 60-month period. That blows my mind.

Casey's story is not just about his physical journey, but also his mental and emotional transformation. He teaches us that success isn't just about setting goals, but also having the right mindset to support those goals. It's about having the courage to take risks and the determination to never give up, no matter what challenges we face. The mindset is a critical component of success, and in this book Casey dives deep on the reasons why.

Casey's story is a testament to the power of grit, determination, and perseverance. He shows us that we too can overcome any obstacle and achieve our wildest dreams. Casey had the courage to pursue his dreams even in the face of obstacles and setbacks.

People with this level of grit don't give up easily. They have an unwavering commitment to their goals, which sets them apart from those who give up at the first sign of difficulty. Having been around Casey it's crystal clear that he desires for you to win as well. He's a great teacher.

I'm in awe of Casey's determination, not just physically, but in every area of his life. Casey's inner strength and the ability to keep pushing forward, even in the face of adversity, inspire me to my inner core. People with this level of determination are hard to discourage. They have a strong will to succeed, no matter what obstacles they face. Casey's determination is unique and contagious.

If you, the reader, are looking to excel in some area of your life, prepare to be challenged at the highest level. Casey's ability to persist in the face of so many challenges seems daunting at first blush. However, Casey masterfully and methodically designs a plan in this book for you to follow so you too can accomplish amazing feats.

If you're like me, I often shy away from hard things. My natural desire and tendency is to take the easy path. That's not the mindset of an Ironman. Even though I'm Casey's life and business coach, I've learned so much from him. Casey is patient, persistent, and tenacious, even when the going gets tough. He's fully aware that perseverance is essential for long-term success.

In *The Power to Change Everything* Casey reveals how you too can overcome significant obstacles and succeed. He starts with Gratitude, which is his superpower. I don't believe we've ever had a session where he failed to show gratitude. Don't hear me wrong, Casey has plenty of areas of his life he is attempting to improve. But in this part of the journey, he's done exceptionally well.

I highly recommend this book to anyone seeking inspiration, motivation, and guidance in achieving their own goals and aspirations. Whether you're looking to pursue a new challenge or simply want to improve your life, this book will help you develop the winning mindset that Casey embodies.

Thank you, Casey, for sharing your incredible journey and for inspiring us all to reach for the impossible.

Aaron Walker
Founder and President, View from the Top

INTRODUCTION

I could hear the ocean roaring in the distance. Like the surrounding crowd of onlookers, it was pure background noise. This moment felt like the ones you see in movies where everything and everyone around you becomes a blur, the camera goes into slow motion and the epic music kicks in.

As my feet pounded on the pavement and ragged breaths heaved from my chest, I braced myself. My legs ached, my lungs burned, and sweat dripped down my neck. The last mile of this race would take an even greater toll from me emotionally than physically. I knew it would; I trained for years to get into the Ironman World Championship. The journey had reached its climax. It was a moment that could go on forever. Even though I still raced against the clock, part of me wanted to slow down and savor it. I wanted to stretch out each second for all it was worth.

We go through different seasons in our lives. For me, this race marked the zenith of a season of tremendous personal change. But all I could feel in the moment was gratitude. As my body performed to its limit, I thought about the people waiting for me at the finish line. My tribe—the people I love deeply, who supported me and watched me overcome one obstacle after another, pursuing a better version of myself. I thought of the ways I'd learned to think differently, and the hardships that forced me to the point of death, until I surrendered and changed my ways. And I was grateful for all of it.

In between these thoughts, I *still* had doubts. I still compared myself to other runners and forgot that I was in the best shape of my life. Imposter syndrome crept in and whispered in my ear, comparing me with the "real" athletes who'd been doing this for years. Their bodies were thin, muscled, and honed to perfection. I felt *inadequate—as* though I didn't "deserve" to be there. I had somehow snuck into their ranks, hoping to go unnoticed—but I'd soon be found out.

"No! I'm running *my* race!" I whispered to myself. "I'm not here to be anyone else." From years of hearing the ruthless, uncompromising voice of my inner critic, I've learned—do *not let those accusations go unanswered*! Talk back to them! Don't entertain the phony narratives … not for one second.

I steadied my breath and pushed on, counting down the quarter mile markers as the finish line came into view. I knew my wife waited there. She volunteered to work the finish line, so she could be the one to place the medal around my neck.

As I rounded the corner, the faces at the finish line became clearer. Several of them held signs, shouted encouragement, and congratulated the competitors as they crossed. I was so overwhelmed by the show of support that a new wave of emotion swelled up, seemingly out of nowhere. Amid the cheers and roar of the crowd, my eyes flooded with tears. The good kind. My vision blurred, but I didn't try to hold it in or save face. Instead, I let it wash over me. I replayed every uncomfortable moment and horrible mistake that led me to the place where I was forced to make this massive change. I savored the feeling of achieving what many—including myself—had declared impossible, just five years earlier.

The tears increased, as I crossed the finish line. I was filled with an impossible euphoria. I was now the witness, the participant, and the driving force behind a new man born that day. I discovered that the end of one race was actually the beginning of another.

Finishing an Ironman involves more than traveling a certain distance in one day. I did it through thousands of daily actions, repeated over several years. Crossing the finish line seemed to reinforce it: True and lasting change happens because you do *several* things differently, for a long time. You take small, consistent steps that lead to massive change and growth. These were the building blocks I stacked, day after day, that led to that glorious finish line.

The finish line of that Ironman was, for me, a moment of good overcoming evil. I overcame enormous obstacles. I did something others said I couldn't do and learned to delay gratification. Furthermore, I allowed God to fundamentally transform my life—in more ways than I can put into words. And in the afterglow, I *finally* understood: *anything is possible.* I realized—if I resolved to reach an "impossible" goal, I could succeed. I could, in fact, alter the course of my own life if I was determined to do so.

I'll be honest, it wasn't easy. It took gallons of sweat, an ocean of tears and a sturdy support network for me to follow through and make the change.

"Change from *what*?" you might ask.

To answer that, let's turn back to the clock—to the moment I almost died.

How It All Started

I was born in 1985. My childhood was rocky (parents divorced, mother remarried) —but I was lucky enough to go to nursing school in my early twenties. While I was in nursing school, I started dating my lovely wife, Brittany, who blessed me with my son, Aiden. I finished my masters in 2009 and began work as a nurse practitioner. I specialized in clinical lipidology and cardiovascular disease prevention. Part of the reason I chose this path came from watching my grandparents' struggles. Many people in my family developed premature cardiovascular disease, and few of them had access to medical providers nearby who could help.

As my career launched, my daughter Alivia was born. I decided to take things a step further—I began studying for a doctorate program. The days were long and full of activity. I would treat patients, come home to my family, and study at night until my eyes failed me. In the morning, I'd start all over again. I was overwhelmed but determined to go to the next level.

Despite a great career, a wonderful family, and the ability to improve myself professionally … things took a turn for the worse on the personal side. I had overloaded myself, and I didn't know how to handle it. Chaos and anxiety took control, and life slowly became unmanageable. To cope, I turned to food.

For me, food was the answer to all life's problems. I ate ridiculous amounts to quell the stress and anxiety. If I felt frustrated, my favorite hot meal would calm me down. If I couldn't sleep at night, ice cream would help. If I was nervous about a diffi-cult patient profile, I could mull it over at my favorite restaurant. Food calmed my nerves and gave me a feeling of being in control. But it came at a price; I gained a ton of weight.

I could see that my appetite was a problem. As my body changed, I became more uncomfortable, inse-cure, and unhappy. I told myself I would exercise, but I had a difficult time changing my diet or adding the gym into my hectic schedule. Because I struggled with confidence, I turned to food even more. This led to "trying" all kinds of quick fixes: smartphone apps, fad diets, you name it. I continued to gain weight, and the possibility of returning to a healthy condition drifted further and further away. Despite my professional qualifications and knowledge of my family's health history, I couldn't stop myself.

It came to a head at age twenty-seven. I weighed 260 pounds. Just one month after I finished my doctor-ate, I awoke one day to find myself paralyzed.

Clinically, I was almost dead—from low potas-sium. When I came to, I could only move my hands, feet, and head. This was rock bottom—the moment I realized how much damage I'd done, and that I couldn't continue the way I used to live. In my mind, I was supposed to have 20 or 30 more years before any serious issues would arise. I knew I had a few bad habits … but it didn't feel like I was running out of time that quickly.

It was clear, though—if I wanted to play with my kids and help them discover the world, I needed to walk again. I didn't want to burden my family or force my wife to have to care for me in that way. I didn't want my children to grow up with a father who couldn't move from a bed or wheelchair. I was horrified by my situation. Enough, as they say, was enough.

I decided to take my life back.

I decided to become a better version of myself.

I decided that I alone would dictate how I lived my life.

I learned you can choose stagnancy and comfort, or you can get uncomfortable and grow.

My journey began that day. Over the next five years, I lost over 100 pounds. I competed in one event after another—events I never dreamed I'd be able to enter. It was a hard journey. It took enormous sacrifice and commitment. But as I crossed the finish line, I can tell you—the ability to move and live life "out loud" far outweighed every second of pain and discomfort I endured.

Today, I own and operate several health and wellness clinics. Together with a dynamic team, we help people change their lives—the same way I changed mine.

I Know What You're Thinking

When I struggled, I experienced every thought you might be thinking right now.

"I've tried it all and nothing works."

"This is too big of a goal; I'll never be able to do it."

"I would love to try, but an expensive wellness plan is way out of my price range."

"I don't have any support, or a community to help me."

I thought all these things and more, too. My goal with this book is to provide you with a different way of thinking. I'll tell you honestly up front: It isn't easy, it isn't simple, and it's not fast. Instead, it focuses on small changes you can make in your daily life to see lasting, long-term improvement. Losing weight isn't a simple recipe you can follow; it's a *mental and spiritual transformation*—you will need to confront a ton of emotions, fears, misunderstandings, and false narratives.

Have you ever noticed that no other creature God made struggles with overeating? Weight loss is a mental/emotional/spiritual problem, as well as a physical one. You have likely thought several of these destructive thoughts, and we need to deal with those things first. If we don't, the tactical things I can teach you will fail. That explains why you've "tried everything" and it hasn't worked. Emotional eating is one of the hardest addictive habits to break—because, like any addiction, it isn't about the food. It's about the *person eating the food.*

Let me repeat that: the food isn't the problem. YOU ARE. I am. We are. Because for human beings, eating is about more than just physical nourishment.

We're self-medicating in hopes of feeling something—anything—that gives us a split second of feeling "better" or "in control." Food offers instant gratification that helps you feel like you're back in the "driver's seat" of your life. No matter how much you weigh or what you look like in the mirror, you will run into the same temptations, even when you succeed! If you don't resolve the *internal* chaos, it won't matter what happens to the chaos on the outside of your body. Only by a bone-marrow deep <u>change of heart</u> will you make serious progress, with lasting results.

My Offerings to You

I can help you make those changes with the concepts we discuss in this book. Gently but firmly, I pledge to help you unwind false beliefs and adopt an entirely new lifestyle—one that will unlock a world of possibilities. (If you follow through on it, you may one day catch yourself asking, "Why didn't I do this sooner?")

This book is made up of eight core concepts:

- Gratitude Is Everything
- Anything Is Possible
- You Can Do Difficult Things
- Be Better Today Than Yesterday
- Learn to Be Comfortable in Uncomfortable Places
- Growth Versus Fixed Mindset
- Small Steps Lead to Success
- Building Your Support Network

Toward the end, we'll talk a lot about the small steps you need to take when it's time to run your race, and the people who need to be waiting for you at the finish line. Eventually, you must lace up your shoes and get out on the road, and there are practical steps that apply. But if you notice, I put them at the *end*, after all the other chapters. Why would I do that?

Once again, if you don't change the way you <u>think</u>, you can't expect permanent changes to how you behave (much less how you look in the mirror). One of my favorite sayings goes, "If you want better answers, you need to *ask better questions.*" It sums up perfectly what I'm about to teach you, because change is only going to happen if you're prepared to question how you currently think—about everything.

It doesn't matter where you are today or how many tactics you've tried. You can be better tomorrow. You don't need a lot of money. You don't have to understand anatomy like a doctor or have all the time in the world. Another saying I'm fond of goes, "You don't need to be successful to start, but you do need to start to be successful." Whatever you do with this book, don't put it down or forget about it. Why should you wait another day, when an abundant life of joy and success awaits you on the other side?

Remember—all I'm promising here is *the truth*. Some days will be hard. You'll have days where it feels like you didn't accomplish anything. Sometimes, you'll feel like a complete failure. It's normal. It's okay. You can acknowledge your feelings, without getting swamped by them. The only thing you must *not* do is give up and walk away. Try again tomorrow, and you'll see—small changes lead to big ones.

It's never too late to begin. If you're reading this book, today is your day. Let's get started on your journey of transformation!

PART ONE:

WHO YOU HAVE TO BECOME

Chapter 1:

GRATITUDE

As a child, my mother never let me forget the importance of gratitude. Even when I wore threadbare clothes and shoes full of holes, gratitude was a pillar in our home. During that time, I remember eating PB&J or ramen noodles for dinner five nights a week and scrounging if we wanted anything else. We had very little.

Growing up, I was painfully aware of how other people had "more" than we did. Even as a child, I noticed. In my early school days, it showed through the kinds of clothes I had to wear and the lunches I ate. Our lack of money continued through high school. My cousins received brand-new cars when they reached driving age. We couldn't imagine receiving things like that.

I remember walking out with them to look at their new cars. The sleek, shiny new paint, the leather interiors, the new car smell, and all the features one could hope for. I recall forcing myself to smile and exaggerating attempts to "ooh" and "ahh" while my cousins talked excitedly about their cars. But no matter how much I tried to be excited for them, it was glaringly obvious to me that I would never have what they had. It broke my heart that I couldn't have something that nice, simply because of the family I was born into. It didn't seem fair.

My mother noticed. She squeezed my hand and leaned to my ear to whisper, "You'll be grateful for this moment one day. You'll see the benefits of gratitude, and how it will change your life."

I *am* grateful—for the hard times. Staying at my grandmother's house because we didn't have a place of our own. Choking down more ramen noodles, for the second week in a row, even though I was sick of them. I'm grateful for how Mom reinforced the value when I was young—when she could easily have become angry herself.

In our house, bitterness, entitlement, and self-centeredness did <u>not</u> fly. No matter how much we struggled, or the obstacles we encountered, we were expected to be grateful. You can hardly blame a struggling parent, unsure how they're going to put food on the table, for wallowing in negativity. And sadly, many do. But Mom refused to do it. Instead, she taught us about gratitude and the importance of seeing the light, even when things looked dark.

Gratitude Is a Catalyst for Change

Gratitude is a powerful antidote to negativity. (How can you sulk or grumble about something you're thankful for?) Gratitude empowers your outlook on a difficult situation. Let me give you an example:

During my competition in Ironman Louisville, I struggled to be thankful. The Ironman is an extremely difficult triathlon; it includes a 2.4-mile-long swim, a 112-mile bike ride, and a marathon on foot—all in the same day. It's something my former self could hardly dream of doing. But it was too late now; there I was, racing in one. I should have felt astounded and thankful that I could even attempt a race like this … but I was in a sour mood.

I had just finished the swim. I jumped on my bike and realized I didn't have my "Bento Box." Ironman competitors pack nutrition to eat after the long swim— energy for the next leg of the journey. Like a kid in school, I suddenly realized I'd forgotten my lunch. I saw the empty space on my bike where the food should have been, and I was *pissed*. I can remember cursing loudly. Without the Bento Box, I wouldn't have food to fuel my body. It felt like I had shot myself in the foot, on a great day with fantastic weather.

My funk continued, even when a volunteer gave me an energy gel. You'd think I'd have changed my tune and been relieved that they offered these gels. But at that moment, I was completely negative. I failed to get all the gel out of the foil packet, and hastily shoved it down into my bag, where it spilled. Ten minutes later, I had slimy goo in the back crease of my knee. I could feel it rubbing in my leg every time I pumped the bike pedals. As my leg went up and down, the stickiness persisted. I was angry, annoyed, and chiding myself. Why didn't I just put it in the trash?!

As I stopped and splashed water on my leg to wash away the slime, it finally sank in—I was angry, and I needed to center myself. I'd worked too hard, for too long, to end up here. My attitude would ruin my day if I let it. So, I took a deep breath, looked around, and searched for something to be grateful for.

This is not "toxic optimism." I'm allowed to have a bad day. So are you. *Everyone* is allowed to have a bad day. When I'm angry, I prefer to verbalize emotion, to help me process it. But after I spill my guts, I know I need to find the silver lining. I need to be thankful if I want to grow.

The gravel shifted under my feet as I moved from one foot to the other. I was *standing*. That alone was an accomplishment; a few years earlier, I was losing the ability to even move my legs, far less walk with a confident stride. I could be thankful my legs still worked. Not only was I walking, but I was running, swimming, and biking. I was *moving*. A man who'd been paralyzed! I took another breath and remembered how far I'd come. I thought of my goals, about the privilege of being alive, and my passion and excitement for the race.

I remembered that my old buddies, "Doom" and "Gloom," weren't going to help me. In over 30 years, they've never lifted a finger to help me once. So, I lifted a finger—the one between my index and ring fingers—to them. I forced my mind to stop its rant. Slowly, through breathing and concentrating, I realized—I was having a *good* race. I'd made great time. I felt good, and I still had the energy to complete the last leg of the trip. In fact, the only things truly *wrong* were external things I couldn't control. I was allowing those external things to dictate my emotions.

Taking one last steadying breath, I got back on my bike. I pedaled hard and let my anger fade as I settled back into the race. I "lost myself" as I continued, focusing my body and mind entirely on the task at hand.

That race turned out to be my fastest Ironman ever.

I didn't allow negativity to stop me or poison the day. Gratitude helped me overcome. It gave me the strength to relinquish control and see the good all around me. I gave myself time to complain —a little. I let my inner critic whine. But after all of that, I stopped and asked, "Is this helping me?" I've learned to demand an answer to that question ... and I've never heard one. The critic goes silent when you confront him.

I Never Said This Would Be Easy

I'm not telling you to ignore negative feelings or pretend they're not real. I don't ignore mine. I just need to process my reactions verbally before I can look at them critically. So, I let my heart speak, even if it's wrong. The only rule is that no matter what complaints arise, I surpass them with gratitude. I may not like how the cookie crumbles, but I can find *something* to be grateful for among the crumbs.

Through my struggles, I learned that you have to *decide* to make lemonade with the lemons you're given. Gratitude is how that's done. You take something sour and hard to swallow, and turn it into something useful. You label what the world hates as "good." You classify your failures as "wins," because of what you learned from them. You drop all charges and accusations against yourself, and trust that you're being *led*—because you are. This journey is never about mere pounds on a scale, or body fat measurements.

You can bet your last penny … it's *always* about what you believe most deeply.

There was a time where I closed myself off from gratitude. I gained plenty of weight, while I lost sight of what my mother taught me. I worked two jobs, my wife worked, we had a young child (and we were still young ourselves). We did everything we could to financially stay afloat, but we weren't getting anywhere. To buy a 2-liter Coke was a heavy lift. On Christmas, I asked my mom for a box of Fruity Pebbles—I hadn't had them in a long time, I craved them, and couldn't afford them. I worried about how to pay for my son's new clothes. And I prayed to God we wouldn't incur any huge expenses, like a flat tire or our heater going out for the winter.

I complained, whined, and avoided my feelings the entire time. I ate everything in sight, causing weight gain and additional stress—which was ironic, since we needed more food, and had almost nothing in our bank account. No good thing we had was "good enough." In my anger and resentment, I began to believe the struggle was too difficult. We deserved *better*. I couldn't believe this had happened. We worked hard, and we still couldn't make ends meet. What was going *on*?!

On a particularly low day, after a long shift, dealing with a hungry child, and my own belly rumbling, I let loose with a bitter, lengthy complaint, from the depths of my soul. I was exhausted from pushing so hard, trying to make life work ... and getting nowhere.

Brittany finally stopped me. Already spent from her own long day at work, she looked up at me with bags under her eyes and said something that stopped me in my tracks.

"Do you realize how much you complain about *everything*?" she asked.

It took everything I had to avoid retaliating. I stifled my next complaint. I shut my mouth and remembered my mother's words. In that moment, I realized I'd formed habits that would have been punishable in my childhood home. I didn't want to be a whiner, but somehow, I'd become one—unable to see the light in the darkness.

Finding my way back to gratitude was a big part of my five-year transformation. It would never have taken place unless I'd learned to focus on the good in my life.

Gratitude Affects Mental Health

There are correlations between mental, emotional, and physical health. They build off one another. The more negativity you take in, and the angrier and more frustrated you feel, the more your body responds, as it says in Dr. Bessel van der Kolk's book, *The Body Keeps the Score*. Some of us avoid this by using drugs, alcohol, or pornography. Others, like me, do it with food. Some keep themselves so busy they can't find a moment to stop and face their pain. There's more than one way to bury your head in the sand and hope the bogeyman goes away.

No matter how far you run from your problems, however, they will catch up with you. They'll shape and control your life, and make it impossible to escape your rut. The old saying is true: "No matter where you go, there you are." If you're miserable where you are right now, jumping on a plane to Hawaii won't change that. You'll still be unhappy when you get there, as well as when you get back.

Ingratitude makes us addicts. It feels impossible to escape—especially when you don't know any other way. Brain science confirms—the neural pathways created by complaints and excuses are so deeply ingrained, it's difficult to stop and reverse or redirect them. You can't undo them without an overpowering habit of gratitude.

Some people "mouth" words of gratitude, as you might "mouth" the Pledge of Allegiance or public prayer—without meaning them. We see cute quotes on notebooks, holiday decor and coffee cups that remind us to be grateful. They decorate fireplace mantles, and caption family photos. But, if you don't stop and get specific about the objects of your gratitude, you'll walk right past these reminders. They're "white noise," ingrained in our culture to the extent that we fail to notice or appreciate them.

I've even seen people use gratitude as the beginning of a complaint! They'll say, "I'm grateful he tried … *but seriously, can you believe…*" or "I'm grateful for what I have! Really I am … *but I wish…*"

Did you ever get a knitted sweater from your grandma for a birthday or Christmas gift, when you wanted a laser sword or a dollhouse? True gratitude is <u>unconditional,</u> just like true love is. It needs to be practiced consciously, without excuses or caveats. You can't just tell yourself, "I'll try to be more grateful" and expect that you'll follow through. You must approach gratitude intentionally, with an open heart. Think about the people and things you're grateful for. Let it sink in. Sometimes I repeat them to myself several times, until I believe the words I say.

The good news is that sincere gratitude has as much of a gravitational "pull" as sincere *in*gratitude. As you improve mentally and emotionally, your body will follow. You'll desire to experience more of the world, to move your body and enjoy everything you are grateful for. Your mental energy interacts with your physical energy, and you experience a rejuvenation.

The key to purposeful, lasting change is to change your mindset. If you change mentally, you can change emotionally, financially, and physically. You can move toward growth. Notice I say *growth* ... not perfection! Remember, the point is to get better, not get it all together. We get the privilege of a lifetime of growth and self-improvement. The project is only finished when we go home to our Father in heaven.

Try Gratitude ... RIGHT NOW

You don't have time to waste. What I'm going to teach you won't work without gratitude.

Read the examples below to yourself out loud. Pause, and think about each one. Think about what they mean to you. If necessary, repeat them 100 times (like I sometimes do) until they feel real. Pay attention to how your mental state shifts after 10 or 15 minutes:

I'm grateful to be alive.
I'm grateful for people who lift me up.
I'm grateful for the ability to improve myself.
I'm grateful I'm still breathing and my heart's still beating.

Do you feel any better when you say those words? The more you focus energy on positive things, the less you'll be consumed by lies, negative thoughts, and false accusations. Marketing guru Seth Godin says, "We don't remember what we see, what we hear, or even what we do. We remember what we rehearse." Being (and staying) grateful requires a lot of rehearsal.

The Critical *Mind* Versus the Critical *Heart*

We're highly critical of ourselves. It's natural as human beings. In fact, if you're reading this book, you've probably encountered the voice of your inner critic. The critic points a finger at your faults and demands that you repeat the accusation under your breath. A critical *heart* is filled with anger or bitterness at circumstances. It sees things as permanent and irreversible. It's quick to get upset and judge others. The critical heart is like a switchblade knife; it pops up in an instant, and it's the weapon of a street mugger. It comes only to steal, kill and destroy.

In these moments, I encourage you to step inside your critical *mind*. Now this is a different tool, more like a surgeon's scalpel. It can cause pain, but the pain is for the purpose of healing the body by repairing damage. Your critical mind helps you ask, "Are these accusations building me up, or tearing me down? Do they restrict and confine me, or do they set me free?" The critical mind can think clearly about bad habits and ill intent, like a detective. It can examine them closely and refute the accusations of the critical heart, because it pays attention to the *evidence* of the damage caused by the critical heart.

Criticism itself is a mere incision from a knife. It can be used to mutilate, or to save someone's life. It all boils down to intent.

Your True Voice

When you become truly and unconditionally grateful, you see the world differently. An old saying goes, "When you change the way you look at things ... the things you look at begin to change." As if, somehow, you went from seeing in black and white to sudden, vibrant color. You notice opportunities you previously missed because you had blinders on. Gratitude is a secret power that allows you to "reset" everything around you.

Of course, with any change of habit, the saying is still true: "Old habits die hard." You will experience the urge to complain. You'll be tempted to think there's nothing to be grateful for. You might come close to giving up the search for things you can appreciate. This is the common condition of being human, and there's no point in avoiding the reality. But when you choose gratitude more often, you'll notice—the opportunities to complain feel more *optional* than inevitable. You'll

start to remember: "I *can* complain here if I want to …
but I don't have to."

When you feel the emotional downward pull, the
key is to get out a *bit earlier* each time. Rome wasn't
built in a day, so don't read this book thinking there's
a "Fast Pass," like at Disneyland. Instead, when you
have a complaint, and you recognize the need for gratitude slightly sooner each time—take the exit ramp as
soon as possible. If your last complaint lasted half an
hour … this time, give yourself 15 minutes. Set a timer,
if necessary. (If you consciously do this, don't be surprised if you reduce tantrums to as little as ten seconds,
or eliminate them completely.) By the time gratitude
becomes your go-to, it feels authentic and effortless,
more natural than forced.

My Joy

For me, I find gratitude by sitting quietly with coffee
in the morning. I block out work, silence my phone,
kill the noise, and avoid external stimuli. I sit still for
10–15 minutes, focusing on all the things I'm thankful
for. This includes relationships, family, God, health,
nature, friends, and the journey I've been on. It's my
way of "stopping to smell the flowers." I take the time
to appreciate things I would otherwise overlook.

I think about things I've previously taken for
granted. I used to hate everything "healthy," includ-

ing exercise, physical activity, and eating correctly. But now, I *cleave* to health; being healthy and taking care of my body are more a part of who I am than bad eating and laziness ever were. I think about my goals and where I want to go next. Neglecting my physical health feels like sinning against God, even for the offer of an occasional donut or "cheat meal." After 17 Ironman races (and another one scheduled at the time of writing), how could I be anything but thankful for how far I've come?

I had to dig deep after the Ironman World Championship. There were no new goals to work for, and no races to compete in because of the COVID-19 pandemic. It forced me to deal with *quiet*—which, in my case, meant dealing with inner pain and uncertainty races had enabled me to avoid. (This is another important lesson with gratitude—when you pass one challenge, you'll face a new one.) The new challenge looked different. It was more *advanced* … I'd built up an "immunity" to the old ones. Triathlons were now pieces of cake … but working on my inner character sounded painful and unpleasant.

If you've ever played video games, you've probably "unlocked new levels." You practice one level until you beat it, and then the game gets more challenging and complex. *But you remain the same heroic character throughout*, which is the secret. In the game of life, you'll unlock many levels—but the person you become when you unlock a new one is very important! In the quiet and isolation of the pandemic, I faced the difficult task of remembering who I'd become—without races, competitions, or events to prove it.

But dig deep enough, and you'll find the memories. When I looked back on my cousins receiving those cars for their birthdays, I realized my mother was right; I had a lot to be grateful for, even then. Today, I'm grateful I was the kid who had to walk or take the bus. I was the kid who had to learn how to earn money. I was the kid who struggled. If I understood how to be grateful, even when everything was wrong, I would remember to be thankful when I stood on the mountaintop as well! And today, that's true: I'm more thankful than I've ever been, and new vehicles and money *chase me*, instead of the other way around.

Change Avoids an Ingrate

I'll say it again: without the firm foundation of gratitude, nothing's going to change. This journey won't work from a place of bitterness and disappointment. Now, I'm not saying you must be 100 percent satisfied with where you are. You wouldn't be reading this if life was working exactly how you'd hoped! But in your dissatisfaction, you need to find *something* to be grateful for. You must *want* change, because your life is a precious gift that's being sabotaged through bad habits and choices. The good news is you can still be grateful for the gift ... AND, you can stop misusing and abusing it. You can treat it with far greater honor and respect and reap a tidal wave of benefits.

I'll say it one more time: find *something* to be grateful for, or you may as well **put this book down**. It won't help you.

In the movie *The Bucket List*, there's a scene where Carter (played by Morgan Freeman) tells his friend Edward (played by Jack Nicholson), "Find the joy." He says this in a letter he sends, while on his deathbed from cancer in his old age. You need to do the same ... even if you're on your deathbed! No matter how deeply it's buried, find the joy. There is *always something good* to be found in every obstacle you face. It can be a lesson learned, growth you experienced, or even something small like sunlight warming your face.

When I can't think of anything to be grateful for, I thank God for breathing. It's His original gift, and if we're alive, we're breathing. Be thankful you're breathing. You'll live to fight another day. You can say to yourself, "Everything sucks, but I'm still breathing. I'm still here, I'm still in the fight, I still have a chance to make it better."

Gratitude is where your journey begins. To build your foundation of gratitude, start by finding three reasons to say "Thank you" each day—to God, your family, neighbors, or co-workers. Take a few minutes to write them down, as you drink your morning coffee (or right before you get out of bed). When you experience obstacles or setbacks, be grateful for them. This is your first great challenge; you must make peace with the present, before you can step into your future.

Chapter 2:

ANYTHING IS POSSIBLE

I t's easier to write the words "anything is possible" *than to do things that seem impossible.* The more seriously you take those words, the more resistance you'll encounter as you attempt to act on them.

I know what you're thinking: You've probably heard the words "anything is possible" a thousand times. Maybe you recoil from them and think, "Anything might be possible for *some* people ... but not me." You may have swallowed the lie that "some people" have all the fun, get all the good genes, the best opportunities, and powerful connections. How can that be? Surely by now, they'd have found the person who hands out privileges and punishments and put that person to death. (In my opinion, they tried … and it failed. He just got up and walked out of the grave.)

I'd argue the reason you hear "anything is possible" so often is that *some people have discovered it's true*, while others have yet to do it. And here's the good news: the reason they've discovered it's true is because they've <u>decided</u> it's true. This is a strange paradox in life—we don't believe it because it's true; it's true, because (and only if) we believe it. The realm of possibility depends a lot on how you feel about it. This has far less to do with fixed realities no one can change.

I don't blame you for your doubts. I never believed this idea either … until the day I decided I was *going to believe it, no matter what*. I recall my own mother saying, "You can do anything you want to," but it never resonated with me. I had no interest in forcing myself to keep trying when I failed at something. Instead, I preferred to decide quickly: "If I don't get it right the first time, it's not worth doing at all, and I'm not going to do it."

When I played baseball with my cousins, we'd split into two teams for a friendly game. Every time it was my turn to bat, I was terrified of stepping to the plate. I was a poor athlete. I didn't like sports or want to play them. Nobody wanted to pick me to be on their team, I never scored any points, and my cousins always expected me to strike out. When I played little league baseball, I'd walk up to the plate and hear muffled whispers. People knew I couldn't play well. They didn't want me there, and I didn't want to be there either.

One time, I hit the ball. I remember my surprise when the bat cracked in my hands as it collided with the ball. It surprised me, and everyone else watching that day. Sadly, this wasn't a Hallmark movie moment, where suddenly I got a lot better, and everyone liked me. In fact, when I did hit the ball, it wasn't even a good hit. The murmuring and underhanded comments paused for a few moments … and then they picked up again on my next at bat.

I just wasn't good. And I didn't believe I could get better.

Self-Imposed Limitations

You know the old saying, "No matter where you go, there you are"? It's not just a saying. My mindset followed me everywhere I went. Whenever something became difficult, it was there in *seconds* to tell me, "Don't bother." I lacked the confidence to believe I could improve through hard work. No one encouraged me or held me accountable, so it felt unnatural to keep pushing on my own.

I lived much of life that way, too—anything difficult was impossible. I dodged difficult conversations and stayed in my comfort zone. If I came up against an awkward or complicated set of circumstances, I'd run away. This became my general approach to life, until my health took a turn for the worse.

As I gained weight, the fat became my identity. I was attached to it, as odd as that might sound. You wonder, "How could someone actually get *attached* to being overweight?" Well, I did. I felt inadequate, isolated, and compared myself with others. My inner critic became loud, like a megaphone in my head: "I'm not good enough! I can't produce results like others can!" I built walls to keep people out, and refused to look honestly at how things were going. I pushed others away and lost support. I thought, "If I keep people at bay, they can't make me feel any worse."

The only time I felt "in control" of anything was mealtime. I used to think, "If you've got good food, who cares what else is going on?" Food brought such comfort. I had control over it. I could modify and use it to shush my feelings of discomfort, inadequacy and loneliness. Eating distracted me from uncomfortable feelings. I could skip sitting with my pain, or process- ing through it. The next mouthful of food felt way more interesting. I felt powerful when I ate—even though it only gave temporary relief. After I finished, I felt bad.

Does any of this sound familiar? All of us have an inner critic, and everyone has something that gives you a temporary "high"—a feeling of control, superiority or simple relief. I've never met anyone who doesn't have something they can turn to if they want to feel better in the moment. These are factory-installed parts of being human, but we end up using them to impose limitations on ourselves.

Which is why I'm here to tell you, one more time: **anything *is* possible**.

Sometimes the hardest thing to believe is the truth: you can make small, consistent changes over a long period of time, including in your physical health. It requires discomfort, but you can do it. You must unravel the "knots" you've tied yourself into, coping with negative emotions. I know nobody wants to hear it … but the reason you're overweight has way more to do with your *soul* than your body. Your condition on the outside reflects how you feel on the inside.

We prefer to think of weight gain and obesity as physical problems, leading many to hope for "magic bullets." People try weight loss surgery, different kinds of diets (keto, fasting, fad diets), or solutions that over-simplify the complex spiritual and emotional nature of human beings. Some go to the extreme and develop eating disorders … but at the end of the day, it all traces back to deep, inner unhappiness. A lack of understanding about life, and how to deal with realities we don't like or understand.

Don't get me wrong, plenty of factors can make change more difficult for some than others. You can have genetics that predispose you to gaining weight quickly. You can face the challenges of mindset and traditions from your family of origin. Maybe you work in an industry where junk food, alcohol, fast food and desserts are set in front of you every day. On a case-by-case basis, I've worked with plenty of people under circumstances like these. But the opposite is also true: you can be a generally positive person, with great genetics and a good family with healthy eating habits … and you can *still* gain a ton of weight, because of inner discontent.

Simple, physical solutions allow us to bypass personal responsibility—and that's why they fail. The simple truth is this: *If anything is possible, and if you can gradually lose 100 pounds with a growth mindset, then you are 100 percent responsible to find the way to make the progress you desire.*

What I Mean When I Say Anything Is Possible

- *"I've tried everything."*
- *"It's too difficult."*

- *"I don't have the time."*
- *"It's too expensive."*
- *"I've always been overweight, and I always will be."*
- *"Eating healthy and working out is miserable."*
- *"I'd rather just be fat and happy."*

I've said all these things myself. They're the opposites of believing anything is possible.

No matter the excuse, or how often you repeat it, that's all it'll ever be: an excuse, that achieves *nothing*. When I say "anything is possible," I mean you need to stop making excuses and start taking responsibility. Responsibility is the foundation of possibility. Once you take ownership of your life, you own it. Only you can make it worse—and only you can make it better!

Rocky Balboa, the protagonist in the "Rocky" film series, is an everyman who gets a shot at greatness: the opportunity to fight the reigning world heavyweight champion. Rocky is a down-on-his-luck boxer, working as a collector for a loan shark. Despite his humble beginnings and tough upbringing, he has a good heart and a strong sense of determination. When he gets the chance to become something more, he jumps at the opportunity and trains hard.

Despite the odds stacked against him, Rocky puts up a good fight and gives the champion a run for his money. In the end, he loses the contest—but wins the hearts of the audience and establishes himself as a true contender in the boxing world. The *Rocky* series explores the theme of *possibility*—the idea that anyone, no matter their background, can achieve greatness if they're willing to work hard and not give up.

This is a great example of how a mindset shift toward possibility can make all the difference.

Another example appears in the parables of Jesus: the faith of a mustard seed. It refers to the idea that even a small amount of faith can produce great results. In the Bible, Jesus says, "Truly I tell you, if you have faith as small as a mustard seed, you can say to this mountain, 'Move from here to there,' and it will move. Nothing will be impossible for you." (*Matthew 17:20*) In this passage, Jesus uses the mustard seed as a metaphor for the power of faith. Even a tiny seed can grow into a large plant, and in the same way, even a small amount of faith can have a big impact in our lives.

If you don't believe you can do something, guess what? You won't do it. If you don't believe you can improve at something, you won't make progress. If you don't believe you can get out of your rut, then you'll remain stuck.

But what happens if you *do believe*?

The next time you face a challenge of any kind, and the inner critic begins screaming at you to give up, what happens if you choose to ignore or over-rule it? What if you say to yourself, "I can do this. It's going to take practice to get better, but I'm willing to work to get where I want to be"? When I got busy running for triathlons, my inner critic got busy running his mouth. But he went quiet when I answered back and said, "Guess what? We're doing it anyway!"

Even now, I still remind myself to focus on possi-bilities. At my first Ironman race, my inner critic threw a fit. Though I'd already lost so much weight, all he could say was, "I'm chubby. I'm going to be slow." Looking at all the toned, muscle-bound athletes there, I felt like every one of them was a judge on a panel to tell I didn't belong.

I confronted the inner critic again. I said, "I may not run as fast as they do, but I can do it. I may not finish in 10 hours, but I *can* finish. My age and weight don't determine who I am. I am still valuable. And if I want to be better, it'll take work and consistency." Don't make the journey more painful than it needs to be. Learn to silence the inner critic and give possibility permission to speak.

Affirmations

You can start this mind-opening process through affirmations.

Affirmations are positive statements you can say to change how you perceive yourself and the world around you. When you affirm yourself, you send new messages to your subconscious mind:

- "I'm worth it."
- "I'm capable of great things."
- "I can do better than I think."
- "God is pleased with me."
- "I don't have to be afraid / nervous / unhappy etc."

Our minds struggle to distinguish between *perception* and *reality*. If you form a habit of affirmations, you can "trick" your mind into feeling and thinking positive. Then it becomes a part of your belief system, stored in long-term memory. Over time, as we continue to repeat an affirmation, our brain accepts it as "true" and starts to act like it. It's a parallel of how negative thoughts influence you to behave; the only difference is that negative thoughts are easy and automatic, while positive ones require courage and conscious effort.

For example, if you repeat the affirmation "I am confident and capable," your brain will start to believe it. You'll begin to act with confidence and capability. You might start to take on new challenges and projects, or speak up when you'd normally keep quiet. Affirmations are reminders that you can do things you'd normally avoid.

Affirmations help you focus on the positive. If you say, "I am worthy and deserving of love and happiness," the message is clear: you are valuable, and deserve good things. Since we all face plenty of "rejection" throughout our lives, affirmations make a huge difference in how we conduct ourselves and where we devote our time and energy.

The Right Affirmations for You

It'd be nice if we could all use the same words and phrases to do this, like a magic spell … but the truth is, affirmations that work for me may not work for you. You can research them on the internet, but I recommend a few "ingredients" for making your own.

#1 Include your goals: Affirm what you want to achieve. Take some time to think about how you want to improve and use it as the starting point. Self-improvement comes in many forms. With this book, you're starting with the *physical—but* if you succeed, you will have transformed your inner being as well. I guarantee it.

#2 Make them specific: Attach the affirmation to a particular goal. General affirmations are good, but specific ones are more effective. For example, instead of saying "I am healthy," you could say "I am healthier this week than I was last week." Do you see how those words focus in on validating your progress in real time? That's how specifics work to your advantage.

#3 Make them positive: How you phrase things can be "negative," even if you mean it positively. Instead of the phrase "I don't eat junk food," try this: "I choose foods that make me feel good and healthy." Define yourself by who you are, rather than by whom you're not.

#4 Make them believable: Make sure your affirmations are believable and achievable. Don't set yourself up for failure by choosing ones that are unrealistic or unattainable. Focus on affirmations you can truly believe in and work towards. For example, you could say, "I will be promoted to CEO one day." But if that's outside the scope of your authority, it could come back to bite you. As an alternative, you could say, "I'm a thoughtful leader others depend on," or "I'm the kind of person people look to for leadership." You don't have to hold a certain office for those things to be true, or possible.

#5 Make them personal: The most effective affirmations resonate with you personally. Think about what truly matters to you and create affirmations that line up with your priorities. Maybe you have a spouse and children you care about deeply, and part of the reason you're on your journey is to be around long enough for graduations, weddings, and grandkids. If this is true, you'd affirm yourself as a great spouse, parent and future grandparent.

Begin Using Affirmations Now

Here are a few steps you can take to make affirmations into a habit:

#1 Set aside time: To make the most of the affirmations, set aside time to repeat them. This can be first thing in the morning, before bed, or whatever time works for you. Cement them in your mind, so you can access them when you run into challenges or difficulties.

#2 Repeat your affirmations: Over and over, until they stick! When an excuse comes to mind, repeat the affirmation instead. If you feel something is impossible, or you want to give up, repeat an affirmation. Did you ever read that children's book, *The Little Engine That Could*? It wasn't just a fairy tale! It's also true. Keeping silent doesn't stop negative thoughts. You already know this, from how your mind normally works. You must get out in front of the noise.

Henry Ford once said, "Whether you think you can, or you think you can't, you're right!" What he forgot to mention is this: "You *will* think one or the other. It's up to you which one."

#3 Be consistent: To see the benefits of affirmations, you must do these drills all the time. Don't worry ... you'll have *lots* of opportunities to practice! The good thing about personal growth is you can guarantee resistance and opposition from your lower self. The rewiring process doesn't happen overnight. Repeat your affirmations every day, whether you feel like it or not. That will prepare you to use them when difficult situations arise. Stick with this for at least 30 days, and you will see the full effects and start a new habit.

#4 Be patient: Remember, change takes time. It may take a while to feel the full impact of your affirmations. Be patient, and trust that they're working to reshape your thoughts and beliefs. Even if this feels silly at first, I promise the practice is worth it. You'd be surprised how many people around you use their own affirmations. In fact, it's hard to find a successful and inspired person who *doesn't* use them. I dare you to try it for a month and tell me whether it has a positive impact.

How I Got Rid of My "I Can't" Mindset

Here are some of the things I made a habit of saying, as I went through my transformation:

"Just because I have a thought, doesn't mean it dictates my emotions and actions."

"My thoughts are like airplanes in the sky and I'm the air traffic controller. I oversee what thoughts 'land' and 'take off.'"

I oversee what I think and feel. I have the power to control my thoughts instead of letting them control me. I could control how I reacted to thoughts the moment I had them. And even if I entertained a thought, it didn't mean it was true, or that I had to act on it.

I started with those phrases because I was used to "mental autopilot." Controlling my thoughts was new. Usually, I'd let negative thoughts derail my day, and end up overeating. Exercising control over my thoughts made it clear: I needed to do away with the toxicity in my mind, so that I could throw away the toxic food in my refrigerator.

President Abraham Lincoln once said: "Most folks are about as happy as they make their minds up to be." If I simply tell you "Anything is possible," you can still choose to ignore or disagree with me, consciously or otherwise. The only way to truly stop saying "I can't" is … to stop saying "I can't"!

Exit: Comfort Avenue

As you go, you'll see an off-ramp at every milepost. You'll face choice after choice to abandon the slow and steady for the quick and easy. The slow road is uncomfortable, unfamiliar, and new. You're learning to understand how to sit and embrace the discomfort. But let me ask you: has the "quick and comfortable" taken you where you want to go? Are you satisfied with the results? How many pounds did you lose on the last bag of Oreos, or 12-pack of Mountain Dew?

Most people choose to be comfortable and in control—the path of least resistance. But if you can "embrace the suck," you find your way out of the maze. You don't have to be stagnant. You could get much more out of life than you settle for. It's just that the door you fear to enter is the door that guards the treasure.

Breaking Free of Impossible

When I took responsibility for my life and opened my heart, I realized the folly of my self-imposed limitations. They feel laughable now, when I look back at how I ruled myself out of activities or used food to cope with unhappiness. My sense of inadequacy and isolation were like a prison cell, where I was both the inmate and the guard. My vocal inner critic kept me from progress as surely as a physical wall would stop me from running.

The old voices come back from time to time, in case you think they're completely gone. When I feel prone to self-criticism, I go back to affirmations and talk through concerns with people who care about me.

Over time, I've grown to trust myself (and others) to counter that voice. Soon, the reality of the situation comes to light, and the critic's complaints lose their power. I'm surrounded by love and support, through a network of people I trust.

As my health improved, other areas began to change as well. I went from working two full-time jobs and struggling, to building a successful business of my own. I went from trying to gain others' approval to accepting that I'm "pre-approved." I helped others make their own mental shifts, so they could recover their physical health. After a while, the "spill-over" effect began to happen for my clients, too. As they improved their physical well-being, other dimensions of their lives improved as well. It reminds me that I'm not special ... which means that if it was possible for me, it's possible for them. And for you.

Today, when something seems impossible, the question is no longer "Can I do it?" Instead, the correct question is, "*How* can I do it?" It's not a "yes or no" decision. It's about the steps I need to take to achieve the goal, and how to get started right away.

Start small, affirm yourself every day, reject your limiting beliefs, and silence the inner critic. Anything is possible for you.

Chapter 3:

YOU CAN DO HARD THINGS

Back in my middle school days, I received constant reminders that my family didn't have the money or resources others did. My peers would get new sets of clothes in the winter, and again in the spring. They walked around wearing the trendiest styles and hottest brands. My clothes, however, were threadbare, my shoes were worn and brown, and I wore the same winter coat several years in a row.

Despite the difference between us, when the time came for students to run for student council, I decided I wanted to give it a try. After all, why not me? I was a student, and the student council sounded fun and exciting.

But other students didn't agree. I remember walking through school, head down, hands buried in my pockets, my shirt thin and several years old when someone bumped into me. The kid standing in front of me wore expensive clothes from one of the popular clothing stores in the mall. I couldn't afford to shop there. He leaned in close and sneered, "You can't run for student council." His tone was haughty, as if I should have already known. I remember feeling my cheeks heat up at his words. I pushed past him and walked away.

I won't lie, those words did make me wonder whether I should give up. But the more I thought about it, the more his words fanned the flame inside. I *wanted* to try for the student council, and just because I didn't come from a wealthy family, didn't mean I couldn't try.

So, I joined the race. I developed a campaign strategy, stayed up late making signs, and brainstormed ideas with my friends. I pushed hard just to prove him wrong. I wanted to show that I did, in fact, have what it took to be on the student council. I would do a good job, even if I didn't wear the right clothes or hang out with the popular kids.

That year, I was elected vice president of the student council. And every year after that, I continued in class leadership.

I Lost My Ability to Do Hard Things

I admire my younger self—he was so full of gumption and self-confidence. But somewhere along the way, I lost this "I can do anything" spirit. I wish I'd kept it, especially when I started gaining weight. Middle school Casey attempted difficult things because he *believed* he could. But adult Casey came to believe difficult things were impossible.

When my son Aiden was born, my wife and I couldn't afford anything. I felt stuck and wanted to shake things up. I found a program called "Couch to 5K" marketed for beginners and decided to try it, but I gave up after two days. It was hard, and I wasn't sure I could do it. I remember saying, "It would be nice to run a marathon, but I can't even go four minutes before I'm out of breath and have to slow down and walk."

My lack of confidence spread quickly to other areas. In our house, if electronics broke, they would often stay broken—because I didn't know how to fix them and refused to ask for help. One time, our garage door stopped working. I had to force myself to do something about it. I Googled, searched, and read every instruction manual and watched every video I could find. Four hours later, shaking from the cold, covered in sweat and dirt and my knuckles skinned and bloodied, I *finally* fixed it. I sat down and wept, because for *once* I'd remembered I could do something difficult.

I'm sure you've faced challenges like this, too. We always face temptation to avoid difficult situations. It reminds me of stories in the Bible of people running from their callings. Jonah was a prophet called by God to go to the city of Nineveh and prophesy against it because of its wickedness. But Jonah resented the people of Nineveh and didn't want to go. So, he tried to run away from his purpose by boarding a ship to Tarshish, the exact opposite direction. God, however, was not deterred by Jonah's attempts to avoid his purpose, and He sent a great storm to engulf the ship. The sailors on the ship were afraid and threw Jonah overboard, where he was swallowed by a large fish. Inside the fish, Jonah prayed to God and repented of his disobedience.

God commanded the fish to spit Jonah out onto the shore, and this time Jonah did as he was told and went to Nineveh. When he arrived, he delivered the message of God's impending judgment, and the people of Nineveh repented. The story of Jonah is a lesson about the importance of accepting and fulfilling our purpose in life, even if it's difficult or frightening.

Another story that stands out in the Bible is the story of Elijah, the prophet. Elijah was called by God to confront the wicked King Ahab and his wife Jezebel, who led the people of Israel away from worshiping God.

After Elijah performed a miraculous demonstration of God's power, Jezebel became angry and threatened to kill him.

Fearing for his life, Elijah fled from Jezebel and Ahab and traveled into the wilderness. He became depressed and despondent, and even asked God to take his life. But God didn't abandon Elijah, and instead sent an angel to provide him with food and water. Eventually, Elijah was called by God to return to Ahab and Jezebel, and he confronted them again. This time, he defeated the prophets of the false god Baal and proved to the Israelites that God is the one true God.

Both prophets eventually did what they were supposed to do, even though the task ahead of them seemed insurmountable. And they did so only after doubting their abilities. It was their faith and determination that gave them strength to take small steps forward until, eventually, their actions saved entire nations.

Difficult things are just that—difficult. But *difficulty* doesn't mean "impossible." It doesn't even have to be a bad thing.

Difficulty Is Part of Life

Avoiding difficulty blocks you from learning and growing. We've all heard the phrase, "Nothing worth having comes easy." I've found this to be true. Everything worth having in life comes with a process to achieve—and the process almost always includes difficulty.

People experience *unique* difficulties, relative to one another. My story probably sounds like "cakewalk" for some, and "hell on earth" for others. Difficulty comes in all kinds of forms: financial struggles, health problems, relationships and so forth. No two people have the same challenges to overcome; what may seem difficult for one person might be easy for another.

However, just because someone else seems to have it "easier" than you doesn't mean they live challenge-free. Similarly, even if you feel like you have it "harder" than someone else, you shouldn't think you're "excused from duty." Instead of comparing yourself to others, you should focus on the unique obstacles in your way, and work to overcome them. By doing this, you can grow and develop as an individual, and lead a happier, more fulfilling life.

If you don't grow, you become stagnant. "Stagnation" happens when a person is unwilling to change or improve. I promise—you don't want to become stagnant. Nobody wants to be mediocre—and stagnation is a great example of mediocrity. This relates to having a fixed mindset instead of a growth mindset, which we'll cover shortly. For now, think of it like a body of water. Stagnant bodies of water, like lakes, aren't safe to drink from. When there's no movement, rot and disease build up over time. Moving bodies, like rivers, are safe to drink from. They move toward a destination, growing faster and stronger until they reach the finish line.

As my life began to turn around, I had to recover the "I can do anything" attitude. It took time, but now I can look at a difficult situation and feel confident I can work my way through it. When new challenges appear in my path, I immediately shift gears and put on my "planning" hat. I look at the problem objectively, and I remember—I need to break it down into small, achievable steps. Just because it's not easy, doesn't mean it's not doable. I don't know what I don't know, *until* I try something new—and usually discover I was missing out on something.

Thoughts Make Your Reality

The first time I went to run, I thought it would feel easy. All day, I thought to myself, "I'm going to go run. This is going to be great."

I wasn't being naive. I knew I couldn't run 10 miles, but I went outside and started running anyway. I made it less than 400 feet before I had to stop. I felt like I was going to die as my breath heaved, and my heart thundered in my chest. I nearly fell over in the ditch because I couldn't catch my breath. All I could think is, "How am I going to make this happen?"

Previously, I would have said, "Screw this, I'm going home." But this time was different. I said, "Okay, I've made it this far. It isn't as far as I wanted to go, but I'll do it again." And I did it three more times that day—for the same distance. The next day, instead of 400 feet, I ran 500 feet. The day after that, I pushed to 600 feet. For six months, I ran in increments like this. Even though I cussed every single day, and kept running up against my own limits, I continued to push myself. I had set the goal of running one mile without stopping or walking—and I wasn't going to give up until I could do it.

Finally, the day came: I ran a mile without stopping. It probably took me twenty-five minutes, but I came home proud of myself. I didn't stop or walk—not once. The non-runner who didn't do anything athletic had started to become a runner!

Once I'd run a complete mile, so many more things became possible. I started to believe, "If I can run a mile, I can run a marathon." The day I came home from my first mile run, I believed it then and there.

If I had the willpower to train and put in the time, I knew I'd make it happen. I still could only run a mile the next day, but it was "too late" for negativity. I was hell-bent on running a marathon. The more I trained, the closer it came to reality. I made it to my first half-marathon, and when I finished that race, I remember thinking to myself, "A full marathon would be a piece of cake!" (It wasn't—but I did it anyway!)

By the time I got to my first Ironman, the stakes were much higher. I was scared to death because my son went to school and told his teacher, "My dad's going to be an Ironman." I wanted so badly for my son to be proud of me like that, but I didn't know if I could finish the race. I knew I could run the marathon portion, but the bike ride, and especially the 2.4 mile swim … I wasn't so sure. I also knew my loved ones would be waiting at the finish line. I didn't want to disappoint anyone who came out to support me.

Before the race, I sat down and said to myself, "Okay, I've put the work in, I know I can do it. Just because I've never done it before, doesn't mean I can't do it today." From there, all that mattered was that I *kept going*. I remember telling myself, "If I don't quit, I can't lose." I repeated that mantra all day.

Crossing the finish line was among the best moments of my life. "Exhilarating" fails to describe it. I had such a euphoric feeling as I realized I'd just done something fewer than one percent of people in the world ever do. And I did it because I believed in myself, even when I knew I would have to work hard. I refused to think of my goals as "impossible." Finally, it had all paid off.

You Can Do Hard Things, Too

I once worked with a client who used to drink three 2-liter bottles of Mountain Dew every day. *Yes, you did read that correctly*. Stopping this habit seemed impossible for her. She drank Mountain Dew with every meal, first thing in the morning, and late at night. Quitting Mountain Dew seemed impossible. But together, we made a plan. I encouraged her to believe she could make a change. Slowly, she began to lower the amount she drank in small increments until eventually, she was down to only one can of Mountain Dew per day!

Labeling things as "difficult" won't do you any favors. Your thoughts dictate your reality. They're powerful, and have a significant impact on your actions, emotions, and how you perceive the world. If you have negative or pessimistic thoughts, you will see the world as a dark and dangerous place. This leads to fear, anxiety, and depression, where you're more likely to make bad decisions and have unhealthy relationships.

On the other hand, if you fill your mind with positive and hopeful thoughts, you'll see a world full of possibilities. Instead of dwelling on how difficult it is to change, think about the small steps you can take today to move one step closer to your goal. If you do this, you'll face a lot less resistance.

There is a reason weightlifters try "one more rep" when they think they can't go any further. It challenges the muscles and promotes growth. When you lift weights, your muscles must adapt to the increased demands you place on them. As a result, they become larger, stronger, and more resilient.

But if you always lift the same amount of weight for the same number of reps and never track your rest time, your muscles will grow accustomed to the demands, and you'll hit a plateau. You'll stop gaining strength and mass. So, weightlifters use a concept called "progressive overload," where they keep adding tiny amounts of weight, and pushing themselves to do "one more rep." They don't go from lifting 100 pounds to lifting 1000 ... they get better by single digits, just like I'm teaching you to do.

If right now you are 150 pounds overweight, it'd be nuts for you to attempt to climb Mount Everest. But that doesn't mean it's impossible for the *next* version of you. Nothing's impossible <u>forever</u>. You can start by saying, "I will be a different person tomorrow than I am today, using healthy, attainable steps to become the kind of person I dream of being."

Stop Saying "I Could Never Do That"

Whenever someone says, "I could never do that," I always come to a complete, dead stop. I reject it out of hand, and I reply, "You can do way more than your mind allows you to do." A person who says "I could never do that" is suffering from temporary, spiritual blindness. If they have mirrors in the invisible world, people who say this would be like Dracula—unable to see their own reflections.

First, you need to surround yourself with people who have the experience to walk you through it and help you learn from their mistakes. You can't "see yourself," so how will you learn from your mistakes? As my grandpa used to say, "If you don't learn from other people's mistakes, you're the stupidest person in the room." You have to find people who have overcome their problems and find ways to spend more time with them.

As things started to change for me, I found help. I leaned into the challenge and sought out people who could teach me. I read books and listened to podcasts by people who inspired me, so I could develop my own plan. I found ways to break my big goals down into tangible actions … and then, *I acted upon them.*

"I could never do that" is always false. Just because your goal is a long way off, doesn't mean you can't even begin. If it takes you several months or *years*, or if it's the last thing you do—make the decision *today*—"No one and nothing will stand in my way, including myself."

Now, let's talk about the framework you need to transform "I could never do that" into "I DID IT." It starts with these foundational steps:

1. Recognize Where You Are

You need to see your starting point without any illusions and name the roadblocks that could pop up. Even if it's uncomfortable, you must stand in the "You Are Here" spot on your map. And if that spot currently has 100 pounds of excess fat, *so be it*. Don't be afraid of those big numbers; they're nothing compared to the power of a determined human soul. But for now, call your situation what it is, without any spin or rose-colored glasses.

Let's say you want to improve your physical health. Give it a name! "Right now, in this moment, I can't run more than 20 yards without getting winded." If you've neglected your health for years, it's unrealistic to start by training for a marathon. So, we're going to scratch that idea, and train to run 20 yards without getting winded. Once you clear that hurdle—only when you've cleared it—can you then add distance or time into the equation.

An honest look in the mirror boosts your self-awareness—a <u>key</u> ingredient of personal growth. Imagine you want to improve your mental health by reducing stress. To do this, you need to stop procrastinating. That is *much* easier to do when you take a good, hard look at the person in the mirror and don't try to sugar-coat or cover up the way you think and do things now.

Here are a few steps to take to understand yourself, right now:

1. **Stop and breathe**. Turn off your phone and other distractions. Concentrate on your thoughts in a quiet and comfortable space. Bring a journal to make a note of what surfaces.

2. Once you feel calm, these **three questions** can help you work through negative emotions and get things off your chest:

    a. What makes you nervous, anxious, sad, frustrated, or angry?

    b. What would life feel like if you were confident, relaxed, joyful, overcoming, and happy?

    c. What stands in the way of you getting there?

3. Be honest when you answer. **Don't judge** your emotions or thoughts … simply express them and let them fall where they may.

4. Now, **write down your answers** to these questions.

5. List **3-5 potential goals** to work toward, to become the person you described in the second question, such as:

    a. Reduce soda consumption by two cans a day

    b. Walk half a mile every other day

    c. Deactivate the snooze button and get up on time daily

2. Break it Down and Make it Possible

Next, you need to break your goals into actionable steps. Find one thing you can start today, to take one step towards one goal.

From this moment, until you can hit the target 10 out of 10 times, you have only one job: *work until you can hit the target, 10 out of 10 times*. If your starting goal is to cut your soda consumption by two cans per day, then you work on that goal until you can't possibly mess it up. A good timeline for this is 21 days. If you can perform the same routine every day, for three weeks, then chances are it'll become part of your lifestyle.

(In case you're wondering, I mean that you cut down your soda consumption for <u>way longer than 21 days</u>! We're talking about a *permanent lifestyle change*, not a three-week fad. But if you can do it for three weeks without fail … you can do it for the rest of your life.)

After you hit the target 10 for 10, you can *gradually increase* your performance. Using the soda example, let's say you've made a habit of drinking two cans of Coke a day, instead of four. Congratulations! You've made a permanent lifestyle change. You dropped your soda intake by FIFTY percent. That's huge! And now, it's time to inform the Coca-Cola company that they are losing another customer. If you could stop drinking two cans of Coke per day … what's to stop you from stopping two *more* cans of Coke?

If you guessed "Nothing," you answered correctly.

And how do we set the next goal? The same way we set the first one: a 21-day sprint to "Coke Zero" —not "Coke Zero" the drink, of course, but <u>drinking zero Cokes</u>!

Why? Because you can, that's why! Because you've already shown the world, "I can kick a two-Coke-a-day habit like a boss." Because if you dropped two of your four-Cokes-a-day in just three weeks, there's nothing to stop you from doing it again. Just like when I planned to run 400 feet, and then pushed to 500 feet—your goals should be small and achievable. The important thing is they feel *possible* and move you incrementally closer to where you want to go.

3. Find Accountability

There's an elephant in the room we need to address— many people dislike the idea of "accountability." They imagine themselves giving authority to someone else to supervise and correct them. That's very different from what I'm talking about.

To truly be "accountable" looks much more like this: *committing yourself to a goal, out loud and in writing, in the presence of someone who cares enough* *to demand the truth from you—a person you do <u>not</u> want to disappoint.*

Everything we associate with accountability—helping to keep track of progress, exercising together or regular check-ins—won't work any other way. If it's a casual friend who doesn't care much about the outcome—forget it. If *you* aren't invested in winning for yourself, it won't work. If your words mean nothing and you don't care about disappointing yourself or others ... accountability is useless.

Having said all that, accountability does give you a greater chance of follow-through. When you set expectations for yourself, you'll stay engaged and motivated, even when things get tough. Good accountability partners provide support and encouragement, as well as question your decisions and behavior. When you face a difficult challenge, having someone to talk to offers space to work through negative feelings.

Here are a few other accountability suggestions:

Join a support group or online community where you can connect with others on the same path. This gives accountability, support, and encouragement.

Consider working with a coach or mentor who can help you to set and achieve your goals, provide guidance and support, and hold you accountable for progress.

Use technology to your advantage. There are many apps and online tools that can help you track progress and stay accountable. Goal-tracking apps like the "Whoop!" band monitor your progress AND connect you with others on a similar journey.

4. Understand "Relative Difficulty"

Remember: what feels difficult today gets easier tomorrow. When I first started to exercise, it felt overwhelming. I didn't know where to start, and every time I tried, it felt like a battle. But as I stuck with it, exercise became more intuitive. Now, it's a skill I enjoy using, the same as if I'd learned to draw or play a musical instrument. This is the truth for anything we do where commitment is involved. At first, it feels daunting and overwhelming. But with time, effort, and persistence, we come to enjoy what once felt like misery.

One thing that's always helped, when I feel stuck, is to remind myself that whatever I'm struggling with now will be easier in the future. The challenges will still be there ... but I will become better at handling them. As the saying goes, "It doesn't get easier. *You get better.*"

When you feel stuck, like you're not making any progress—remember, it's your race. Your only "opponent" or competitor is your *lower self—the* person you've allowed yourself to become. What other people do, or how quickly they achieve things, has nothing to do with your race. If you need to stop, take a breath and wait until your head clears … do it! Things will get easier in the future. Keep pushing yourself and don't give up. You can achieve more than you think.

5. Start Moving

When it comes to personal growth, remember—progress is a *journey*, not a destination. Like any journey, you will make mistakes. It's better to mess up on the way to becoming who you want to be, than remaining stuck as you currently are.

Are you the same person you were five years ago? Of course not. The real question is, "Who do you want to become, in five years?" One way or another, five years from now, you *will* be a different person. If it's going to happen anyway, why would you want to leave it to chance? There are things you can do immediately to go in the direction you truly want to go.

Once you break your goals into bite-size chunks, you have one job: keep moving forward, no matter what. It's way easier to say than do, I know—until you do it! Once it becomes a habit, you'll wonder why you didn't do it sooner.

And when you mess up, remember your "why." Remember the person you want to become. Repeat your affirmations. Stay connected to your accountability partners. Find and build relationships with people who challenge and encourage you. Remember that difficulty is relative.

Because you *can* do hard things.

Chapter 4:

BE BETTER TODAY
THAN YESTERDAY

Working in healthcare, I often talk with people discouraged with the amount of weight *they have lost*. Not gained … *lost*. I sit in my chair, with the client across from me, excited to check in on their progress—and I can see it on their face. Disappointment. At least twice a week, somebody tells me, with resignation in their voice, "I lost a little bit of weight, but it wasn't as much as I wanted. I suppose 'slow and steady wins the race.'"

I can feel their disappointment, like a Jedi Knight who can feel another's anger. They've turned their negative emotions inward, beating themselves up about their "lack of progress." They might put a positive spin on their words, but their body language tells another story. They refuse to celebrate or accept their growth. It's like they want to "beat me to the punch" of criticizing themselves.

Have you ever met someone who makes fun of themselves before anybody else can? It's the same idea. They expect others to reject and ridicule them, so they try to be the first person to say it! Patients in my office have the same problem. They see others further along their journey, so they talk this way to avoid the discomfort of someone else pointing it out.

These comments typically come from patients who have just started their journey and lost 15-20 pounds at the most. When they see other patients in our community group who've lost 70 or 80 pounds, they feel condemned, like their own progress doesn't matter. But they fail to see that the clients who have lost eighty pounds have typically been on the journey for months, or years! It doesn't matter; the new patients mercilessly read themselves the riot act.

People feel tempted to see a page in someone else's book and wish they could have the same results. But they don't realize or appreciate the *chapter* of the story they live in. We don't always see the full context—especially when we're so close to the action. If my clients had to watch each other's stories on *video*—from beginning to end—they'd see the full price paid by the veterans. Instead, the only thing the new patients focus on are the results they notice on one given day.

Which is why you need to learn that every step forward makes you better today than you were yesterday. And to accept this progress, you must get out of your own way.

Have you ever heard of the "lizard brain" response? It refers to how our minds quickly and efficiently process threats. By attuning ourselves to potential danger, we have a greater chance of staying alive. This process, of paying special attention to the negative, is hardwired into us. When we have a negative thought, we receive a surge of activity in the critical thinking area of our brain, so we can assess the threat. And we *keep* thinking about it, until we feel certain that we've neutralized the threat. This can trap us in cycles of negativity. It's helpful in a survival situation, like a jungle where tigers lurk behind every bush. But our minds don't always remember the difference between *real* threats and *imagined* ones. We must consciously switch off these alarm signals, and it takes practice to do so.

When I hear these comments from discouraged patients, I remind them that losing weight slowly helps you to keep the weight off in the long term. Why? Because you get used to a different *lifestyle*, which causes lasting change. "Crash diets" frequently result in explosive weight gain after a couple of months because there's no lengthy period of adjustment. So, the person who loses 20 pounds on a crash diet goes right back to their old eating habits.

So, can you take the risk that gradual change is a *blessing*, rather than a punishment, for your past choices? Can you stay focused on the idea that God is being *kind* to you, by going slowly? Do you see how your heart and mind may have become too critical … and maybe it's time you set their comments to the side? I promise you this: Learning to love your journey beats any destination you could choose. If you need to lose 100 pounds and you can learn to love yourself through losing just five, you'll learn to value being kind to yourself much more in the long run.

Progress Over Perfection

When a child learns to walk, everyone coos and cheers over their first steps. Our parents' hands hold us up, so we don't fall and hurt ourselves. We receive praise when we take a first step, and then two, followed by three with the support of a sofa or table. When we finally take steps without the support of anything around us, we get a new round of applause.

Little children have intense, constant support systems. Each small discovery or moment of learning brings praise and celebration. But as we grow up and become adults, our support system deteriorates. Schools teach, model and reward perfectionism. The workplace too, because (we think) perfection leads to promotions and profits. In our homes, mothers and fathers struggle to be "perfect parents," while working stressful jobs. Perfectionism surfaces in little things, like the disappointment from ruining a recipe or staining a shirt with bleach. Life seems to be *designed* to turn us all into perfectionists, and shames anyone who rejects or rebels against the model.

Perfectionism is everywhere in our culture. Maybe that's one reason we see more anxiety and depression these days, especially among teenagers. We've lost sight of the truth: Perfection was never the goal. Progress is the goal.

Mark Twain once said, "Success is a journey, not a destination." As a recovering perfectionist, I keep it top-of-mind. My phone's background reads "Progress Over Perfection," so that I don't forget it. I suspect many of you struggle with this concept as well. We demand more of ourselves than we have to give and refuse to enjoy the journey. When we focus too much on the destination, we miss out on the beauty of the journey. Our goals become the objects of our perfectionism, which means that anything except achieving them equates to failure. (And even if we achieve them, we immediately discard them and ask, "Now what?")

We have *got* to stop believing this! Making mistakes or coming short of your goal should *never* equal "failure." If you made progress, you made *progress* … period! You are different from who you were yesterday. Even what we call "failure" really means "winning," so long as we learn or grow from it.

People often reject their own progress through fretting about the past or the future. They might dwell on some glorious moment in the past, such as when they were an athlete in high school, or life was one big party. Or they think of some glorious moment in the future when they'll "arrive" (i.e., they'll achieve perfection). Instead, we need to focus our attention here and now, and stay in the moment. There's no such thing as "arriving." None of us will ever achieve perfection.

You'll always deal with unexpected challenges. Remember how I forgot my Bento Box lunch at the Ironman race? Things like that will happen to you, too. You must learn to work through and overcome them. Every attempt at growth gives us *more* to work on and improve. We think, "If I could just _____, I would be happy." We look at people with greater health or wealth and assume they don't have any real struggles. We think their lives are perfect, and they have everything together.

That's a mistake. It's false! Those people have stressors and things to work on, too. It just doesn't *seem* like it to you because they are in a different stage of their journey, where the problems they face aren't obvious to you. But that doesn't mean they don't have them!

If you pin your happiness on a destination or goal, it won't be long before you put a negative spin on progress and give in to perfectionism. Instead, find ways to appreciate the journey—because that is where you'll learn the most about yourself. Even the slightest progress you make today counts as growth from who you were yesterday.

Wax On, Wax Off

Every now and then, fiction does a better job of describing reality than reality does. Have you ever seen a movie with a character stuck in a set of circumstances where there was no way out ... except to become better?

One of my favorite movies is *The Karate Kid*. Daniel LaRusso, the main character, moves to a new school where he gets bullied. He meets Mr. Miyagi, a karate master who agrees to mentor him. Early on, Miyagi requires Daniel to spend long hours waxing cars, sanding wooden decks, or painting fences. Daniel gets frustrated; he isn't sure Miyagi is truly training him. He thinks he's being used for manual labor. When he confronts Miyagi about this, the karate master shows him how the moves from waxing, sanding, and painting have trained his body in the basics of karate. From that moment on, Daniel realizes Miyagi *is* training him—with small steps that lead to big results.

At first, it's easy to sympathize with Daniel's complaints. There's no time devoted to kicking, punching, blocking, or sparring … So how could he be learning karate? But when Miyagi reveals how the work has sharpened Daniel's reaction time and instincts, it's our turn as the audience to change our minds. Now we realize—*far more* was going on, than originally met the eye! In only a few long days of super-repetitive work, Daniel's karate skills have grown more than they would in three weeks in a dojo!

When my clients are unhappy with their progress, I hear a few phrases that sound like Daniel when he confronted Miyagi:

"This has been a waste of my time."
"This goal is impossible."
"I'm not seeing results fast enough."
"What is the point, if things aren't changing?"
"This isn't working."
"I didn't lose as much as I wanted to."

I've had these thoughts myself. I learned to counter them with a firm conviction, that *I will grow* from the experience. At the beginning of training, I might say, "Man, this is gonna suck! I haven't felt like this in a while. I'm about to do hard things and push myself. I must embrace the suck." If my attitude that day is sufficiently bad, I'll repeat it to myself out loud, *as I run*. It's how I remember that even if something feels uncomfortable, I can still do it. Even if I don't feel the desire, I can still put in the work.

Affirmations play a big role here. You need to remember who you are—especially when you're over halfway through and the pain starts to amplify. This is the process of developing your personal bandwidth. If you listen to the lies and accusations in your mind, rather than your affirmations, you'll stop believing. What's true in the light is still true in the dark—it's just harder to feel. So, bring yourself back to the truth: "These goals are 100 percent achievable. Anything is possible. I can do hard things. I will learn and grow from this. I will get one step closer to achieving my goals."

Incremental change is hard to notice if you don't feel like you're winning. If you have to squint to see progress in the mirror, or on the scale, you'll feel the temptation to throw your hands up. If you don't see the progress on the outside, remember—there are *huge* changes happening on the inside. Internal changes also show results on the outside—they're just more subtle than a loss of two waist sizes. I see and hear them all the time! Changes in posture, body language, eye contact, tone of voice, energy, enthusiasm, and word choice all qualify as changes. When I see these changes happening, I know it won't be long before the extra pounds are gone, just like the negative emotions.

1 Percent Goals

Sonia Thompson says, "Setting the bar too high can demotivate and discourage you from ever getting started." To avoid this, we need to learn to create 1 percent goals.

When I say "1 percent goal," I mean "something that takes you one step closer to your vision today than you were yesterday." It means reducing a marathon, for example, into a one mile run without stopping. To make measurable progress, your 1 percent goal could be running a little further each day—from 500 feet to 600, and from 600 to 800, 800 to 1200 and so on until you can run all 5,280 feet in one mile.

One percent goals should be things you can fit within your existing schedule and energy levels. It shouldn't take up large chunks of time or feel overwhelming. At the same time, it's also about being *gracious* with yourself: "If today, I set a goal to run 600 feet instead of 500, but I only get to 550 feet before I have to stop … that's *still* progress." Sometimes, even

1 percent goals can be ambitious. You may even need to set "one tenth of one percent" goals!

You can learn a thing or two from the video game industry, when it comes to setting 1 percent goals. Most games include small, easily achievable goals which over time build your avatar into an epic hero. In fact, this is part of what makes video games addictive. Much like the dopamine hit you receive when playing a video game and you unlock a new level, smashing a 1 percent goal gives you confidence and keeps you hungry for more.

And it's not just video games. Successful tech start-ups use the "scrum" process to take things a step at a time, constantly course-correcting, until they grow and become corporate giants. Athletes start from ground zero and train to operate at peak performance, by training in increments. Writers start with simple ideas before they can write entire sections and tell page-turning stories. Everybody starts somewhere, so it's time to part ways (permanently) with the idea of "overnight success." It doesn't exist.

As Zig Ziglar said, "You don't have to be successful to start, but you do have to start to be successful."

How To Set a 1 Percent Goal

Now that we know what a 1 percent goal is, let's talk about how they can work like compound interest. Do you have a 401(k) or retirement plan? They operate on the same principle. We covered breaking goals down into smaller segments with target dates. Now, let's dig a little deeper, and create an example set of goals, so you can see what they might look like. We'll keep breaking it down until we get to 1 percent goals. Your 1 percent goals should apply to each segment of the bigger picture.

Bigger Picture: Run a Marathon in the Next Twelve Months

Segment Goals:

- Run a mile without stopping after 2 months of practice.
- Run 7 miles without stopping after 4 months of practice.
- Run 14 miles during one session after 6 months of practice.
- Run 22 miles during one session after 8 months of practice.
- Run 27 miles during one session after 10 months of practice.

First Step: <u>Run a mile without stopping after 2 months of practice</u>. If there are 5,280 feet in a mile, that divides into 88 feet per day over 60 days. So, if you start very small—88 feet, less than a third of a football field—your first day will be over quickly. By Day 3, you want to try for 352 feet—a little longer than an entire football field. If you double the amount of feet every day for 60 days, you'll end up at one mile.

- Day 1: Run 90 feet without stopping
- Day 2: Run 180 feet without stopping
- Day 3: Run 360 feet without stopping

Now here's what you **don't** see happening—your body's getting used to running every day! Your mind is getting used to "the suck." By the time you're in Weeks 7-8 of this phase, your mind and body will be very used to running. They won't hit the panic button when you pick up the pace. So, even though it might feel a long way off—by the time you run your first mile, *it won't feel like a mile*. If anything, it'll feel just like running 176 feet felt on Day 2—a little further, but not by much, from what you did on Day One. It'll be even easier if you took time after Day One to celebrate and acknowledge your achievement.

That's the most important detail: Once you complete your 1 percent goal, *celebrate* your progress! Remember how little time it took, and how easy it was. This is what causes your mental attitude to shift. The next time, you'll be less inclined to feel fear or resignation, and more likely to feel confidence. Give yourself a pat on the back. You took a step towards a massive change in your life!

"Celebration," in most people's minds, usually involves spending money or throwing a party. It's important you recognize the win, but spending and parties are risky. Remember the example of video games? If you've got youngsters at home, you've probably come across their Fortnite dances like the "Floss" or the "Griddy." (Look them up, I'm not going to print them here.) My point is, the video game heroes do a little "happy dance" when they unlock a new level, and then they move on. NFL receivers do the same thing … and then it's back to work. The *parties* are for when you win the Super Bowl.

How to Satisfy Your Soul with Just 1 Percent Progress

I know it's difficult to appreciate 1 percent progress when what you really want is 100 percent. I have wrestled with my limitations, too. Let me give you an example:

I ran pushing my cousin, who has cerebral palsy, through several half-marathons as I progressed through my journey. It's something I deeply enjoyed doing. On one occasion, however, we competed in a race on a bitterly cold day. Temperatures were in the twenties, with a wind chill in the teens. Even though others in the race had been kind and offered to help push him, I didn't appreciate them, nor did I take their help. Why? Because I was angry.

Here is how the conversation went in my head:

As the miles began to tick, I felt like trash. The air was cold, my lungs were heaving, and I thought, "This sucks!"

I looked at my watch, and realized I was losing speed! I berated myself and thought "Move your ass! You gotta go faster!"

We turned a corner on a beautiful, oak-covered Southern street with old plantation homes. I began to catch up to the main body of the race, until we hit a hill. It was the only hill in the race. I thought, "Put your head down, shorten your stride, and get up this hill!" I decided to run full-force up the slope.

We finally crested the top of the hill, where I had even more trouble catching my breath. I realized the mistake I had just made. My lungs felt shredded, and I thought, "I'm gonna pay for that!"

Even though I pushed through a lot of mental blocks in this run, I forgot to take time to appreciate my progress. I was conquering more milestones that my former self would have refused to try. None of this occurred to me until we were running a straight shot through the middle of downtown in the last mile of the race.

Only then did I realize—my negative thoughts were taking over! I paused, bringing myself back to the present moment. It was time to change out the soundtrack in my head.

I said to myself, "Casey, there were some sketchy times in the middle of the race where it looked like you'd fail, but you are exactly where you need to be. You did those hard things, and you're still moving forward! Now, you need to focus on *this minute* of the race. You can't change what's behind you, or what's far out in front of you. But you can affect what's right in front of you, in this moment."

As I pushed my cousin close to the finish line, we came to a stop. I scooped him out and helped him settle into his crutches. He walked across the finish line with me, and we cheered like it was going out of style!

It took that entire race for me to remember to affirm my progress. Imagine how much more confident I'd have felt, if I'd made a point to recognize and appreciate the ways I handled the obstacles when they happened! Your soul will only be satisfied with a 1 percent goal if you take time to *appreciate it*.

All those 1 percent moments add up to who I am today. All the small victories stacked up, and now I understand—I have "failed my way to success." I can look at photos of myself back then, and see how I've become two different men, in every sense of the word.

This is the world of progress that 1 percent goals, recognition and appreciation open for you.

Dealing with Dismissal

Once you set your 1 percent goals, watch out: The most dangerous obstacles to your momentum are dismissal or diminishment of your progress—whether by you, or from others.

I hope it doesn't happen for you, but unfortunately it is a reality. When we work to improve ourselves, the people around us may become doubtful, or even discouraging. If someone ever dismisses your progress as "too slow," or tries to shame you for taking small steps, I advise you to take a deep breath, reject what they say and remove yourself from the situation.

You worked hard for your progress. If someone pooh-poohs your excitement or effort, that's their problem. Change the subject, or leave. Don't share the topic with them again. You and I need encouraging and supporting voices in our corner—if haters are gonna hate, let them hate alone. Don't give them an audience.

If their unpleasant words hang around, ask yourself, "Is listening to this over and over again *helpful* to my journey, or not?" If the answer is, "No" (and it almost always is), let them go. Reject them, refocus, and reframe the situation. Remind yourself why small goals matter. Reflect on the true progress you've made so far. No destructive criticism!

But remember—you can block your own progress, with how you talk to yourself. Even in the best shape of my life, running the fastest Ironman I ever ran, weighing the least I'd weighed since 7th grade, I *still* felt captive to the size of my waist. Body image issues require a higher-level mindset shift. I could not allow the negativity that once lingered rent-free in my mind to diminish my progress.

You can ruin your progress as much as a jealous friend or family member. If you feel yourself doing this, put a stop to it immediately. Use your affirmations and remember it's the *progress* that's important. No matter how small.

Small Wins Stack Up

As you achieve your 1 percent goals, count each one as a win. These wins will stack up and build your confidence. You'll face challenges with a new attitude. You'll smile more and feel happier and more fulfilled. Things that previously felt impossible will suddenly feel possible, as if a switch flipped in your mind. After a while you'll realize, "This won't even take 10 seconds, why have I been putting it off?"

As they finish my program, patients often tell me, "I never knew this was possible, but I trusted the process, put in the work, and believed that what you said was going to happen, would happen. And it did!"

I don't see why it should be any different for you.

PART TWO:

WHAT YOU HAVE TO DO

Chapter 5:

LEARN TO BE COMFORTABLE IN UNCOMFORTABLE PLACES

Change is new and uncertain. It goes against everything you've accepted as normal—which is why you need to expect to feel uncomfortable. Expect it, embrace it, cheer for it, label it positively—*whatever it takes*, to avoid slipping into a victim mentality. Even if you're physically comfortable, say, sitting on a yacht, in a vacation home, on a fluffy couch or curled up in bed—you can still be stuck in your comfort zone and feel miserable. I've done it myself, and seen it happen to many clients.

Without the willingness to stretch and feel uncomfortable, you'll get stuck in a different kind of discomfort. It's the kind where you stagnate; where, when faced with the idea of tackling change, you pull away and do nothing. You're already stressed about life in general, so you think, "Adding hard things onto my plate won't do any good." Instead of making changes, you stay in a rut of disappointment, anger, and resentment at your lot in life. It turns out that no matter what you choose, you're going to end up uncomfortable.

Change involves discomfort, but so does ignoring the need for it. You must choose which "hard" you prefer. When people notice the choices I make about what to eat, they sometimes say, "That doesn't look fun. It looks unpleasant." Maybe … but you know what's also unpleasant? Feeling powerless against your own appetite. Feeling like you "have" to eat, for the sake of eating. After years of being enslaved to my appetite nearly killed me, I decided I'd rather be able to say, "No" to it.

Fear of discomfort is what people feel, when they say they want to wait for a "perfect" time to change. They say, "I'll wait till after the holidays and do a big New Year's resolution." Or "I'll work out before summer, so I can have a beach bod." Well, summer comes around every year like clockwork for you, just like it does for me … do you see a beach bod in the mirror? By the time everyone's ready to go to the beach, people are busy making new excuses, like "I've been too busy, I'll do it once things settle down at work." They kick the can down the road because the idea of taking responsibility for themselves is *uncomfortable*. The timing has nothing to do with it.

My near-death experience involved every excuse in the book, as I pushed away meaningful change … until the day I lay in a hospital bed, on the verge of losing everything. I understand how easy it is to settle for what's comfortable. But the truth is, "comfortable" won't lead you anywhere but where you already are. I don't think you'd have read this far if you were happy and fulfilled right now.

Slip Into Something *Less* Comfortable

Your habits, relationships, and environment all reinforce your comfort zone. Which means you need to take a close look at who and what surrounds you, to figure out what needs to change.

Relationally, you need people who challenge you, call out your excuses, and tell you what they honestly think about your decisions. People who will hold you accountable, encourage and believe in you. People who've walked the same road you're on. They celebrate your victories and understand the hardships you face. They inspire you to do what you say you'll do— like go to the gym or make better choices about food. They use more positive than negative language … but if they can't make you see the light, they'll make you feel the heat.

Now, I don't mean you cut people off and never speak to them again. I never rejected my friends. But if I went with them to eat, I went prepared. One time, I went to a gathering where I knew ahead of time there'd be a lot of unhealthful food, so I brought steaks and steamed broccoli. My friends ate what they ate, while I ate my steaks.

There may, however, be times where you need to remove yourself and not be "as connected" to certain people. Especially if they badmouth your progress or tempt you with foods that undermine it. If you don't have the self-discipline to handle the presence of certain people, you need to withdraw. Food is addictive, and peer pressure is powerful. Sometimes you must call a spade a spade and walk away.

You should also look at your "go to" foods, especially comfort foods. Macaroni and cheese, ice cream, and anything else that gives you the "warm and fuzzies" (so you can avoid frustrating emotions) need to be removed from your diet. They are addictive because they bring comfort and instant gratification. Everybody wants happiness, success, and results *right now* without giving anything in return. I'm challenging *you*—become the exception to the rule! Flip the pyramid of minimal effort and maximum gain, and pour your maximum effort into *minimum* gains, so they add up over time.

Here's another uncomfortable truth: your feelings don't dictate your actions. We often think once we become "successful" or "healthy," we won't have bad feelings anymore. Wrong! Even the most motivated and healthiest people in the world get the urge to hit the snooze button, overeat and over-indulge themselves. The only difference is that successful and healthy people *push through* those feelings. They don't allow themselves to be ruled by their emotions. They decide to go against what feels "comfortable" into the "uncomfortable." Fear of discomfort makes zero sense! Remember, as I said at the beginning of this chapter—*you're going to be uncomfortable, one way or the other*. The only real choice you have is over what kind of discomfort you prefer.

According to the New Testament, Jesus spent the last night of his life in Gethsemane, a garden located on the Mount of Olives in Jerusalem. While there, he prayed to God, saying, "My Father, if it is possible, let this cup pass from me; yet not as I will, but as you will." (Matthew 26:39)

No one would disagree that Jesus was anxious and distressed about what was to come. But even when he faced the most difficult and uncomfortable moment of his life, Jesus still chose to follow God's will and submit to discomfort (extreme discomfort, in his case). This story shows how we can find strength and comfort in being obedient to God, even amid pain and sorrow. Jesus' prayer in Gethsemane also demonstrated his humanity and vulnerability. Despite his identity as the Son of God, he still experienced fear and doubt, just like we do. But he refused to surrender the power to *choose* how he responded to his emotions and his fate.

The doubt you feel is natural. Everyone who's walked the road you're on faces it. But it's safe to say that if Jesus could accept being betrayed, arrested, beaten, falsely accused, wrongly convicted, humiliated, spat upon and crucified … you can start with two less cans of soda per day. Or with whatever small change you need to make.

Changing Habits Isn't Enough

I began this book with gratitude, belief in the impossible, embracing hard things, and becoming better today than you were yesterday. It's my way of explaining that before you make the physical shift, you must change how you think, feel, and speak. If you don't, you may as well be playing "Chutes and Ladders" with your future—you'll get two steps forward, and then go ten steps back, depending on how you roll the dice.

I had to approach situations differently once I was committed to the journey. I could no longer give up, throw a tantrum, quit, make excuses, or complain. Instead, I had to be patient, quiet and persistent. It's not enough to change a behavior; you also need to change how you *think* about the behavior. As the Stoic philosopher Marcus Aurelius once said, "If you are distressed by anything external, the pain is not due to the thing itself, *but to your own estimate of it*; and this you have the power to revoke at any moment."

Habits are driven by underlying thoughts and beliefs. If you don't address how you think about the things you do, the habit will persist, no matter how you attempt to change it. If you procrastinate, for example, you should ask: "Why do I procrastinate?" If you don't think about it at all, that's a telltale sign you've *delegated* your thinking … it means someone or something else is thinking for you. And that's not good.

Don't misunderstand—I'm not suggesting you need to sit on the floor and ask yourself, "Why do I put on my left sock first, followed by my right sock?" You're a fully grown adult, and you don't need a nanny. We're talking about habits you turn to when things are unpleasant or uncomfortable. If you've gained a ton of weight and feel miserable, isn't it at least worth asking *why* you keep doing the same thing over and over, expecting a different outcome?

Flipping the Puzzle Pieces

Discomfort never goes away completely, but it does get easier with gratitude, affirmations, and laser-like focus on 1 percent goals. When I prepare for a grueling triathlon, I break it into the tiniest pieces I can. I know ahead of time—I will be running, swimming, and cycling. I want to compete in each leg of the race as fast as possible. For that to happen, I plan my training in months, weeks, and days. Once I'm clear what I need to do each day to prepare ... I don't think about the triathlon. I only focus on getting to one mile, two miles, ten miles, and so forth. Then, as soon as I reach that goal ... I stop! I forget all about the triathlon and celebrate: "I ran two miles today!" That's *it*.

You could compare this to assembling a 5000-piece puzzle. If you've ever tried one, you know—it can't be done in an hour. There is a process puzzlers follow: sort the pieces, put the outer border together, and pick sections to build the interior based on distinctive features and patterns. Can you complete it in a day? Maybe—but few people do. It's usually done little by little, with the pieces coming together until the picture becomes clear. At some point, that puzzle is finished, and everyone can see the beauty of it. I encourage you to think about your transformation the same way.

Why Our Brain Tells Us to Stop

Have you ever left your lawn sprinklers on "Auto" in the wintertime? The human brain can be like a sprinkler system. It does what it's supposed to do … even when it's not supposed to be doing it.

Though discomfort from exercise and dietary changes aren't truly dangerous, our minds tell us to stop or avoid uncomfortable things. Whether it's because we aren't used to it, or we associate the activities with negative outcomes, we receive the "Stop!" message. If you're new to exercise, your brain may send this message because it's not used to the discomfort. If you had a negative experience in the past (like my story of being unable to hit the baseball), you associate it with discomfort or embarrassment, and your brain goes into protection mode.

Fight or Flight Response

When we feel threatened or uncomfortable, our brains go into "fight or flight," a natural response to stress. Stress hormones like adrenaline cause physical sensations: your heart rate increases, you sweat, and your muscles tense.

Many of my patients learn how helpful it is to *communicate* with your body. The body doesn't truly know the difference between running away from a wild animal versus running to lose weight. It only knows whether something is comfortable or uncomfortable. This is your chance to "talk" to your body, and tell it, "Everything's okay. We're going to be fine. There's no danger here. We're doing something new, and you're just not used to it yet."

You might think this is strange, but here's another one that threw me for a curve: *Your body communicates with your soul.* It's been doing it for a long time. It tells you when it's hungry, thirsty, tired or in pain. Do you think it's pure coincidence that every time you get tired, you also get irritable? Or how when you're in certain emotional states, it also tells you things like, "Go get some ice cream!" Your body has a way of "remembering" the last time you felt badly, and it prompts you with memories to go and look for whatever "medicine" you used last time to get out of it.

Genuine Pain Avoidance

Some of my patients ran into *genuine* pain when they started their journeys. If there's one thing more dangerous than a patient with low motivation, it's a patient who's motivated beyond a reasonable doubt.

Are you trying to run ten miles, when you haven't run in ten years? If your goal is realistic, I recommend you try to accept pain as part of the experience. But if you need to lose 100 pounds and you want to start by running a triathlon … you need to go slow at first and run in small increments before you attempt anything more arduous. Otherwise, you might end up with something more serious—injuries, being hospitalized or possibly death. Be kind and patient toward your body. It's not ready to handle things like that just yet!

Past Experiences

Past experiences and associations are another big category. We associate activities and situations with different feelings. If we had a negative experience with something, our brains warn us to steer clear of it, to avoid repeating the discomfort or pain. It's natural to hesitate or fear repeating something unpleasant or painful. But the good news is that it's also possible to quietly tell your body, "It's okay. It's different this time. Thanks for the warning, but you can relax and breathe. We're going to be fine."

Personally, I talk through my past experiences with my supporters. In their presence, I acknowledge my feelings as valid … AND I refuse to allow them to stop me. As Martin Lloyd-Jones once said, "Have you realized that most of your unhappiness in life is due to the fact that you are *listening* to yourself, instead of talking to yourself?"

I love that quote. It gave me inspiration for a new mantra: "Talk to yourself. Don't listen."

Lack of Familiarity

When we do something we've never done before, anxiety and stress flare up. And guess what? You can soothe and encourage yourself about this one, too. Yes, I'm giving you permission to walk around your house and talk to yourself. You can say things like:

- "This is unfamiliar … but I'm going to be okay."
- "I don't fully understand … but I'm going to continue working at it."
- "I don't know how long this will last … but I know I'm going to get better by doing it."

How to Convince Your Brain to Keep Going

Whether your goal looks like reducing Oreo Cookies from fifteen per day to ten, or replacing Coke with Crystal Light, it will feel uncomfortable at first.

Once, during a few 3-hour runs to prepare for an Ironman, in blazing Mississippi heat with 80-90 percent humidity, the voice of negativity crept into my head. My feet pounded the pavement, sweat dripped down my neck. The unforgiving sun beat down on me and the humid air made everything more difficult. I felt sticky from the moment I stepped outside, and it only worsened as I exercised. I began to think, "It's too hot to train!" and "I can do this tomorrow."

I was uncomfortable. My clothing was rubbing in all the wrong places. My mind wasn't dialed into the run. The only thing that got me through it was visualizing the finish line of the Ironman. I wanted to finish. I *had* to hear the announcer say, "Casey Elkins, you are an Ironman!" To clear my tempting thoughts, I envisioned the announcer shouting those words again and again to make it through that run. I had to remember why I was training in the first place.

Ayelet Fishbach, a professor of behavioral science and marketing at the University of Chicago and author of *Get It Done*, said, "You might only learn to love your class, workout, or new job after trying it a few times. When people can positively spin otherwise negative cues—reappraise their discomfort as a sign of achievement—those cues become more motivating."

To convince your brain to keep going, you must remind yourself *why the pain is worth it*. As Simon Sinek says, "Start with 'Why.'" You didn't start your journey because life was sunshine and lollipops, and you were completely happy. You've got family and friends who love and care about you. You've got a former self to prove wrong. You've got a score to settle with pain and discomfort. You've got emotions that are like schoolyard bullies, and you need to set them straight. You've got a God to live for, a community that needs you and a life you've secretly dreamed of living.

Make the Discomfort Feel
Uncomfortable Around YOU

When you're uncomfortable, it's a good time to get curious. Leaning into discomfort means intentionally facing and embracing the uncomfortable feelings, instead of running away. But you can't confront those feelings if you don't know who or what they are.

When I hear the voices of discomfort, I'll sometimes say things like "Who are you?" or "What are you trying to get me to do?" It's remarkable how these voices want to stay so hidden and anonymous, like internet trolls or identity thieves. One or two questions like that, and they disappear faster than they showed up. This might sound ridiculous … but remember, *those voices are making intelligent human arguments.* They're not barking like hound dogs. They're talking to you in English, and they're using your own internal voice to persuade you by repeating what they say. Who says you can't talk back to them?

Next time you hear the voice whispering, "This can be over if you'll just compromise," fight back! Say it out loud: "No! No compromises! I'm not stopping! I'm not giving up! I'm not quitting!" You'll be amazed how quiet it gets after you say it … especially if you do it in a public place!

(On second thought, don't do it in a public place … I'm just saying.)

Find Support

The Bible reminds us that "Two are better than one … and a threefold cord is not easily broken."

Have you ever tried to fight two or more people at once? It's impossible! Yet when people try to make a change, what do they do? They lean on personal will-power and pit their vulnerable souls against their inner pain and discomfort. That's what we call "stinkin' thinkin'." If you haven't figured it out, you're already divided on the inside. The way out of sabotaging your own success is *to do it in community*, with people who support you, cheer you on, hold you accountable and throw a red flag when you're wrong.

I love it when I get into the wrong frame of mind, and my supporters throw the red flag. They refuse to listen, and their outrage amps me up! If I start getting down on myself, they interrupt and say, "Casey, I don't want to hear it! You're an Ironman! Snap out of it and get to work!"

Choose Your Hard

Learn to find comfort in "discomfort, fulfilling its purpose."

When things are uncomfortable and I am going through the "suck," I keep my eyes locked on the growth occurring. I embrace and claim the suck as my own. I know I'm moving toward a better version of myself. I know that self-discipline will help me get what I'm after. Whether it takes a week, a year, or 10 years, it's a process I trust. To me, pain and discomfort are *gifts* clear signs I'm on the right path.

I used to seek out instant gratification. But today, if someone offers me instant gratification, I run *in the other direction*. If someone holds out a "get rich quick" scheme or a weight loss pill, I completely turn my back on the offer. I go and seek out the *challenge*, where growth is guaranteed. Through this I've learned to deal with uncomfortable situations that go way beyond exercise and nutrition, because I choose to walk through conflict instead of away from it.

I noticed this when I dealt with a disagreeable person in my circle of friends. Now that I was accustomed to facing conflict, I asked, "Am I contributing to this problem somehow? If so, what can I do to change?" I was open to the idea that I was partially (or even fully) responsible, and their discomfort provoked them to behave the way they did. Maybe I'd said something offensive, without intending to. Whatever it was, I was open to working on it.

Eventually, I took a step back from this person. Sometimes, people respond negatively to you, and the only appropriate thing to do is to make a clean break. But I was glad that I paused and looked at the man in the mirror. I've grown comfortable being uncomfortable, and so I extend more grace and patience to others, rather than point fingers. Even if you only bear one percent of responsibility for a situation, you can create a huge positive ripple effect by owning your part.

When uncomfortable and unpleasant realities surface, I accept them wholeheartedly. To me, they're just opportunities for growth, in disguise. "Comfortable" realities, on the other hand, tell me to be on my guard against stagnation. When I discovered I could overcome the uncomfortable and stand tall on the back side of it, I found something far more valuable than a smaller waist size. I found *peace*. Peace deep in my soul, like a dead calm on the Gulf of Mexico, not too far from where I live. (It beats a hurricane any day.)

I want to assure you—if you stick with it, remain grateful, affirm yourself and hold on tight to what you believe—you'll find way more than you bargained for. Hang in there. Don't give up. It'll suck at times, but it sucks less if you learn to appreciate the suck.

If it wasn't *hard*, it wouldn't be *worth fighting for*.

Chapter 6:

GROWTH VS. FIXED MINDSET

When our family struggled, change felt impossible. No matter the issue—financial, physical, or mental—we had a hard time moving the needle on *anything*.

I thought I'd got suckered into the "rat race" everyone talked about when I was growing up—normal life as an American adult. Adulthood, which I'd been in such a hurry to reach as a child, was here, and it was anything but fun. *This* was the "American Dream" I had been promised as a kid?! Did success really mean shackling myself to work, paying bills and facing one responsibility after another without a break? It never felt like I was making progress. Life threw one thing after another to discourage me from moving forward.

I felt disappointed, frustrated, and dissatisfied—to the point of exhaustion. Was this how the rest of my life would go? If you've ever heard sayings like, "This is as good as it gets" or "This is just the way it's going to be," that's how I felt about it. There was no light at the end of the tunnel. I believed the man I was in those days would be the same man I am today, and forevermore. I remember sitting on my couch, as my children cried and my stomach rumbled, angry about another overdue bill in our mailbox. At that moment, I thought, *"This can't be what life is supposed to be like. There has to be a better way."*

Looking back now, I can see I lived through those days from a fixed mindset.

Have you ever felt like this? When you have a fixed mindset, you feel like a victim of circumstance. Life "happens" to you, rather than the other way around. It darkens your mood and robs you of clarity. You struggle to move forward, and you feel like change is impossible.

Some of us turn to vices to cope with this hard-nosed reality. People become dependent on substances, hobbies, relationships—anything that helps them ignore reality in the short-term, while racking up higher costs in the long run. The cycle feels permanent and inevitable. We believe we're just unlucky beings who will fail to find success, the way others do.

What do you do to get out of this rut? Where's the secret door? How do you get out of the maze? What does it look like to escape this dungeon? The truth is there's a lot of "better" available to you. But it's inside you, waiting to be called forth. The problem is that you must work for it—and so long as you remain in a fixed mindset, you can't work hard or long enough to get it.

Stuck In the Middle With You

In childhood, fixed mindsets earn rewards based on *performance* rather than *effort* (growth mindset). It usually comes through praise and reinforcement by teachers, parents, and other authority figures, a carrot-and-stick routine that gives you a prize in exchange for achievement. Carol Dweck's *Mindset* is a thought-provoking and informative book. I gained a *ton* of insight from her stories of how mindset shapes our destiny, for better or worse.

Dweck said that a fixed mind believes its intelligence, potential, tolerance for pain and other spiritual qualities are finite. If this sounds like you, then you probably say some of the things I've mentioned before: "This is as good as it gets," "That's just the way it is" or "I've always been this way, so I'll always be this way."

A growth mind, meanwhile, believes its abilities and intelligence can be developed and improved through effort and learning. If you're in growth mode, you probably say things I've learned to say: "I can be better tomorrow than I am today," "This is just one page in the story," and "I'm not the man I was five years ago; therefore, I will be a different man five years from now, too." Dweck's book confirms it—your mind is the most powerful tool you possess to turn *weakness* into *winning* and *pain* into *power*.

How do you handle it when you hear the voices of parents, teachers, and authority figures? Do you still feel like life is a *binary* game, where you either win or lose? How's that working out? When you win, do you feel like you've finally "made it"? Or do you soon slip back into feeling miserable? When you lose, do you feel like you've learned something? Or do you feel like you've just proved what you believed all along—that you're not worthy? Most of us received some very unhelpful messages as children. It's time to walk away from them.

One of the biggest "fixed" ideas that stands in your way is fear of failure. This fear holds people back from exploring and discovering their God-given abilities. Culturally and socially, failure has a bad rap. Deep down, we know that failure helps us learn—but that's no use in a culture with overdeveloped image-consciousness, where achievement is glorified, and failure is a byword. It's a cultural joke to acknowledge a failure by saying, with a hint of sarcasm, "You get an 'A' for effort." But in the story I'm living, failure is *good*. Effort is everything! We need to shift into a growth mindset and embrace both failure and effort. Forget achievement, and seek *growth*, because growth IS achievement!

And then there's fear of criticism—internal and external. Start trying to grow, and watch the long knives come out. If you aren't careful, you'll provoke people around you who would otherwise be pleasant and friendly. Like a bombshell rocking a beautiful new dress down Main Street, you can expect hisses and whispers. You've poked the bear! You're moving ahead of people who want to stay mediocre and miserable. If there's one thing that bothers people with a fixed mindset, it's people with a growth mindset. Get used to it; haters gonna hate.

Your inner critic should also go berserk, just like mine tries to during an Ironman. But remember—*you can talk back to that voice!* Use your affirmations, and remember to ask that voice to reveal its intentions toward you:

"Are you trying to tell me I'm better off not even *trying*? Who do you think you are? Where is this conversation even leading us? When are you going to stop pointing your finger and lace up your shoes and help me finish this race?!"

Recognizing a Fixed Mindset

"I can't do it, I've tried everything, nothing works."

"This is too hard. It's impossible for me."

"This is just how I am. There is no changing it."

Here we go, every day. The clients walk into the room, looking at the floor with a melancholy tone in their voice. Though I do everything I can to welcome them, their answers to my questions are short, and they lead to short, closed statements that sound like courtroom verdicts.

When this happens, I change my strategy. I start by asking "Yes" or "No" questions that focus on their mindset: "Do you think you can get better?" or "Do you have hope for a better future?" If they say, "No," I "lend" them my hope for the week. I say, "Here. If you can't come up with any hope of your own, take mine. You're going to be better, and remember this conversation when things get tough."

Hope and faith don't seem close by when you're demotivated. Many people would rather keep up negative self-talk, procrastination, avoiding decisions, and wallowing in their hopelessness. I know I did, for a spell. But that's also why I offer hope to others; if someone else believes in you, what are you going to say? It's like turning down Jesus when He said, "He who comes to me, I will never cast away." The keyword is "never." If He's promised never to cast you away … why wouldn't you go to Him?

Don't surrender to a fixed mindset! Author Morgan Snyder once said, "We can never have the full measure of what God gives us here on Earth … but we settle for a *lot less* than we could have!" Why should you get the "leftovers" in your faith, career, relationships, or health?

Developing a Growth Mindset

I love watching *Big Hero 6* with my kids. It's a movie about a young robotics prodigy named Hiro Hamada. After the untimely death of his older brother, Hiro becomes the leader of a group of high-tech heroes who use their skills and technological expertise to fight crime and injustice.

Growth mindset is one of the main themes of the movie. Hiro initially sees himself as a disaffected, directionless teenager. Soon, however, he embraces his potential, using his intelligence and creativity to make a positive impact on the world. Hiro's "big wakeup call" comes when he realizes an invention he created (which his brother encouraged him to develop) is being used for the wrong purposes. It jolts him out of his depressed state, and he gathers a heroic group of friends to battle his enemy, Alistar Krei.

Wakeup calls like this are integral to change. Everyone has a "rock bottom" they face—even if it's coming within inches of death, like I did. It's a moment where you take a step back and realize how far away you are from where you hoped to be. You give yourself time and space to acknowledge the damage you've done. Every client serious about transforming their life has a moment like this.

Knocking on heaven's door was my first wake up call. The second came when my wife asked, "*Do you know how much you complain?*"

At first, I thought, "I don't complain *that* much!" But the longer I denied it, the truer it rang. Her words carried more weight than my body did. I couldn't shake them. Eventually, I realized—they rang like a bell because she was right. I complained, all day, every day.

Coming from a childhood where gratitude was a rule of the house, it shocked me to realize how negative I'd become. Life was one big melting pot of pessimism—mental, physical, emotional, spiritual, and financial gloom. Everything I thought about turned bitter and sour. But in that moment, when I caught a glimpse of myself, I was horrified. Of all the things I'd ever wanted to become, a *whiner* was NOT on that list!

As I thought about it more, I remembered a lesson I learned in nursing school. One day, while teaching us to administer needles, one of the instructors said, "There are hundreds of thousands of nurses across this planet. They're not special. If they can do it, you can do it. You must *work* to make it happen; it won't come to you on a silver platter."

I began to insist to myself, "I *can* do better." I had the freedom to grow and act. I could control my situation—or at least my response to it. If I wasn't satisfied, I could do something about it. I could change how I thought about things. This was the moment I shifted back towards gratitude and believing anything is possible. I abandoned my heart of stone and exchanged it for a heart of flesh. Only then could I begin to crawl, walk, and run on the long road back to redemption.

Addressing the Internal

In the beginning, your mindset boils down to a simple decision. I can't put it any simpler than that. You can't undo the past, but you *can* declare, "From this day forth, I DECIDE to live differently. I'm not going to think the same way I have in the past. I'm not going to be ruled by my feelings in each moment. I get to decide how I respond to things—not my emotions, my habits or anyone or anything else. *I* decide."

As I recovered, I started applying decisiveness everywhere. I became intense and intentional about the smallest of changes. I focused on how I spoke. If I said something the way I used to speak, I'd stop and publicly retract what I said. I stopped spending money recklessly and took control of my finances. I tricked myself into going to the gym by buying clothes I was excited to wear. Every time I dropped a waist size, I rewarded myself with a wardrobe upgrade.

Addressing internal roadblocks is a challenge. There were days I *made* myself get up. My alarm would go off at 4:30am so I could get to the gym by 5:00am, and my body *refused* to move. I had to trick myself by saying, "After you brush your teeth, you can go back to bed." But once I was up, and my teeth were brushed, I forced myself out the door, like Darth Vader, "altering the deal" as I went. Eventually, going back to bed was no longer an option. Today, it's unthinkable; I haven't done it for years.

Things got hard at the gym. I would run on the elliptical machine for 15 minutes, take a 15-minute break to catch my breath, and get back on for another 15 minutes. Some people set goals, but they don't leave room for their own weaknesses. For them, it must be *all or nothing*. No! A small step in the right direction is 100 times better than no steps at all, just because you struggle to do it perfectly. A growth mindset means *some* effort is better than nothing, even if you can't execute it the first 50 times you try it.

Internally, you'll battle pressure to surrender to your comfort zone by remembering why you have to make these changes and affirming your choices. Managing your attitude toward the journey is difficult. If you remain "negative" about what you're doing, you might see a physical change—but you'll rot on the inside.

Another great strategy I found, that's become popular in the last few decades, is "gamifying." Instead of perceiving yourself as "burdened," you can learn to treat the occasion like a challenge. You can begin to ask, "How hard can I push myself?" This spills over into other areas of life; you can "gamify" everything—money, fitness, relationships. You can play this game to win, and whenever you fail to hit a specific goal, you can adjust your methods and try again.

Addressing the External

I also encountered external resistance. I ran head-on into negativity from other people. They'd say, "This isn't going to last … Casey's just talking … he'll stick to it for a little bit then stop … these changes won't be consistent."

I don't blame people for thinking this way. They had watched me try enough fad diets and different work-out programs to know that I usually gave up after it got uncomfortable. This time, however, I blocked out their voices. I told myself, "To hell with everybody, burn the ships, we're going full speed ahead!" I realized at that moment—what others say doesn't matter. I used their doubts to *fuel my progress*.

Food was another matter. People at work brought junk food to the office to share. I had to train myself to walk away. Pharmaceutical reps would bring cinnamon rolls and Lebanese food for everybody, plus extra to take home. I finally got to a point where I said, "No, thanks. I'm not trying to be ungrateful or disrespectful. You can bring this for the office, but today it's a 'No' from me." I knew *one bite* of a cinnamon roll would turn into eight. I had to build up the willpower to control myself.

And let's name the most awkward one—becoming vocal and assertive, when people try to put you down, diminish what you've done or sound like they're "concerned" about your health. Save this one for extremely rare situations ... but be prepared to tell someone, "I don't want to have this conversation with you," turn around and walk out. The last thing I'd want for you is to end a relationship ... but I've had to do it a few times. Some people just don't take the hint, and you can't let them be the voice that stops you from pursuing the life God has for you.

Looking Through a Fixed Lens vs. a Growth Lens

If you enter a competition of any kind, you'll find people with both lenses: a fixed lens and a growth lens. I see it all the time when I run triathlons.

Fixed mindset athletes look at the competition anxiously. They worry they'll do poorly and relive all the times they've struggled in the past. They get frustrated when they encounter roadblocks, so their performance suffers after their first challenge. No matter where they place, they end up disappointed with their scores (including first place).

Growth mindset athletes arrive at the competition determined to perform their best that day, no matter what. They feel secure in the work they did to prepare and look at competition as an opportunity to improve. They don't care about ribbons or medals as much as others, and they feel more excited about the improvements they make, from one event to the next. If it's their first competition, they remember the progress they made to get to this point (even if they don't place anywhere near the top).

Many of my patients come to me with a lot of weight to lose on the outside, and even more on the inside: a deeply fixed mindset weighs a spiritual ton. When I work with them, I teach them that this is a *lifestyle* change, not a three-week crash diet. It's a marathon, not a sprint. I help them switch to a growth mindset and cultivate a love for the journey instead of a frantic race for a result.

Un-Rut Yourself

Remember the story with my cousins and their new cars? A fun, sleek, car would have made an exciting gift when I was a kid. But looking back, I'm glad I didn't get one. I feel more gratitude for things I've worked for than I do for things that were given to me. Gains I receive from my efforts are longer-lasting and more meaningful.

Today, I know that better than I ever have—and yet, I *still* fall back into thinking with a fixed mindset. And so will you. Switching your view of the world to a growth mindset takes years. Even in your healthiest moments, you'll still find yourself slipping into the fixed realm. You'll deal with imposter syndrome and doubt your abilities. You'll put up your own roadblocks when you're faced with the possibility of change. You'll assume things that aren't true.

Negativity is the first clue that you're slipping back into a fixed rut. If you're regurgitating old complaints, or feeling insecure, address it quickly. Call in your support network and tell them what you're feeling. Step back and ask yourself, "Which mindset is in control here?" Remember, if you're in growth mode, your next question should go something like, "How can I fix this?" or "How can I cooperate and get better in the process?"

For me, I talk to myself *out loud*. I don't care if I look crazy, I talk to myself. But by the same token, I don't *listen* to myself, which is helpful. Only by hitting the "Mute" button on my inner critic, can I work my way back to a growth mindset. It starts with a mental shift, expressed by a change in language. My patients learn to abandon the phrase "I have a weight problem," and exchange it for "I *had* a mental and emotional problem." They learn to say, "That was then, this is now. That is not who I am today. It's certainly not who I'm becoming tomorrow."

My patients go from the deepest, darkest dungeons of despair … to the penthouse suite with the skyline vista. They experience total life transformation. Many start off down, depressed, helpless, beaten, and needing to lose over 100 pounds. By working with the strategies and tools in this book, they transform into a new person. They become lean, muscular, athletic, and they get to do things they thought were impossible.

Remember, you'll be glad you did this! The best part about the mindset of growth is that when you've grown, no one and nothing can take your maturity away from you.

So don't stop now. Let's grow together.

Chapter 7:

SMALL, CONSISTENT STEPS LEAD TO SUCCESS

Without understanding the power of small, consistent steps, I'd never have made it this far. Going from "obese" to "Ironman" would've failed if I'd tried to do it all at once.

Audacious goals like losing 100 pounds feel overwhelming. Most obese people feel like that's what they must do. It's why they experience multiple failures. The task seems out of reach. Once you reach a certain weight, you feel as if you're "too far gone." Phrases like "I've let myself go" ring out like smoke alarms, alerting you that even if you escape with your life, the house probably won't make it.

I certainly felt this way when I started. If you've tried everything and nothing's changed, it's a sign you haven't broken your journey down into small enough "bites" that you can win. So, when I work with clients, this is often where we start—in the smallest, most granular details.

What "Small Steps" Really Means

When I talk about "small steps," some people think "First, run a marathon. Then run a triathlon."

No! That's not what I mean at all. We must think much smaller than that.

Let's say your goal is to lose 50 pounds. If you start with steps like completely cutting out sugar or going to the gym every day, those are too big; you might as well not even try. Steps like these require you to make significant lifestyle changes, and they deprive your body of a substance you're used to. It's a rude awakening, and when people are emotionally vulnerable, it's going to trigger a backlash. It's almost like asking an alcoholic to stop drinking "cold turkey."

I remember trying to cut out sugar. I experienced such powerful cravings that I "broke," and ate sugar again within 24 hours. I was addicted. My body convulsed under withdrawals and fought with my mind every step of the way. It wasn't something I could just "turn off." I had to *slowly* change my diet, be kind to my body and lead it gently toward better eating habits.

The same goes for the gym. Forcing yourself to attend the gym every day when you're not in the habit will feel like drinking from a firehose. Not only are you losing an hour or two of your day, but you're also waking up earlier and making your days longer. You're asking more of your physical body than you have in a *long* time. It will put up a huge fight in response.

Another hang-up for me with the gym was self-consciousness. When I was obese, I behaved like a hermit. I reached a point where I didn't want to be seen in public, and I'd avoid being photographed. If I had gone to a gym full of fit, athletic people with muscle tone, low body fat and cardiovascular endurance, I'd have run away in shame. If that bothers you like it bothered me ... don't do it.

When I say small steps, I'm talking about *tiny* ones. Don't clear out your refrigerator and pantry and refill it with foods you hate. Instead, you can gradually reduce your intake and make smarter decisions.

If you drink eight sodas a day, drop it to six a day for three weeks. Then you take another step: drink only four a day, for three weeks. When it comes to food, pick one meal a day that you *always* eat—usually dinner—where you can *reduce* portions. You still eat all your favorites; you don't "restrict" meals by any means. You simply reduce your portions by 50 percent. You eat, and then you wait 30 minutes. If you want something more after that, you go and get it. Build and hold that pattern for three weeks, before you attempt the next level.

Most people discover, after waiting thirty minutes, that they don't need to go get more. They're surprised to find that they're full, with only 50 percent of the portions they used to eat. If you eat until you feel full, which some describe as a "stretch of the stomach," you've eaten too much! You shouldn't feel uncomfortable after a meal. You should feel satisfied and energized. Gradually reducing portions allows you to continue eating your favorites. There's no need to deprive yourself. You simply learn to enjoy your food in moderation. Do you see how this is different from a crash diet?

When many of us were children, the adults in our lives told us to "clear our plates." Whatever they heaped onto our plate, we felt obligated to finish—even if we were full, or not very hungry. It became our unconscious habit, so that the thought never occurs to us— *we don't "have" to clear our plates*! But you can use this unconscious habit to your advantage. If you serve yourself smaller portions, you'll feel full. You'll make meaningful changes *and* get the "attaboy" feeling that comes with clearing your plate. We're talking about doing something you've always done … just doing it a little differently.

This is how you meet yourself *where you are* … so you can eventually get to where you want to go.

As you think about your "small steps," it's important to understand *why* you turn to certain foods or drinks for comfort. Let's take soda for example. Not everyone gets hooked on soda for the same reason; some do it out of habit, others rely on caffeine, and some remember a favorite grandparent drinking it. To understand why a certain food or drink has such a hold in your life, you need to dig into the details of how the habit formed in the first place. This is helpful when you decide which small steps you're going to take. You can center them around the root cause, instead of the surface-level symptoms.

Maybe you drink soda because you think, "I need the caffeine to function." You used to stay up late, and always felt tired in the morning. Maybe you were an insomniac, or you had a baby who needed you day and night. You started drinking soda to get by. The reason for your habit should inform how you manage it. Whatever the reason—it's okay to tell your body, "That was then; this is now." You can start going to bed earlier, because your child is grown up, or the insomnia's gone away— the only problem is, your body never got the memo. So now, it's time to teach your body the new reality.

For me, eating was emotional. I managed my feelings through meals and snacks. I ate when I was sad, angry, frustrated, or tired. I chose my small steps to address the feelings differently, instead of depending on food. They took the forms of "affirming my way" through anxiety, and expressing gratitude as a response to my negative emotions.

Drastically changing your lifestyle *without* understanding where your bad habits come from is like trying to fill a strainer with water.

A woman I worked with insisted she couldn't lose weight. She had tried *everything* and was convinced there was something wrong with her body. When I introduced this concept to her, she was skeptical, but she eventually agreed to give it a try. She still ate what she wanted, but simply had smaller portions. Eventually, she came back a few pounds lighter and exclaimed, "I can do this!" Because she didn't have to adjust what she ate, but simply *how much* she ate, she was more energized and motivated than any fad diet could have hoped for.

Sometimes, your eating habits are tied to how the people you live with handle food. They might not be receptive to your changes. Some patients have told me, "My husband and kids don't want to eat healthy food." Other families can be obnoxious and rude, mocking their spouse, child or sibling who wants to change things. Several of my patients used this as an excuse for avoiding change.

It's true—you can't control how others respond to your new choices. But you *can* control how you respond to their responses! Each person has their own expectations, feelings, and preferences. You can't let their thoughts or opinions hold you back from making your own changes. You must find a different way.

It might take a little extra work but remember—we're talking about *small steps*. Let's say you normally have a can of Mountain Dew with lunch, mid-afternoon snack and dinner—for a total of three cans each day. If your small step is to drop your Mountain Dew consumption by 50 percent, you could switch to pouring half a can into a glass for lunch, and drinking the rest of it mid-afternoon. Then, you could pour another half-glass at dinner, and save the rest in your refrigerator for the next day's lunch. Do you see how this works? You're still drinking Mountain Dew at lunch, mid-afternoon and dinner. But you've also cut your consumption by 50 percent!

Maybe you're thinking, "Sounds too good to be true"? Many of my clients felt the same way, at first.

But think back to a time when you celebrated a small win. Maybe it was doing your dishes before tackling household chores. Maybe it was buying supplies for a new household project. Do you remember that feeling? The excitement of something greater to be accomplished as you carry out the first small step?

That's the feeling we're chasing.

The Hero's Journey Is Full of Obstacles

You may not reach your overall weight loss goal in a year. It may take you two years or more, depending on how much you need to lose. And even when you reach your ideal weight, setting goals should remain part of your life, so that you keep the weight from coming back. Remember: *lifestyle, lifestyle, lifestyle*. Forget "diets." We're making a new YOU. Right now.

If you feel like you aren't moving fast enough, remember: *you are moving*. Life is meant to be "lived in the day, and measured in the decade," as Morgan Snyder said. Struggle and discouragement are parts of the human experience. You are not a machine; you must expect failure, and plan for it. Now, this doesn't mean you need to fake happiness when you fall off the horse. Disappointment is a natural reaction. But you do have to remember your value, despite your mistakes. The goal is to last a little longer than you did the last time you stumbled.

In fact, mistakes and obstacles are so common to our experience that we create stories, movies, and TV shows about it. The heroes of these stories overcome flaws, setbacks, and challenges, on their way to happy endings. The most popular structure is "The Hero's Journey," which follows the process of an ordinary character, who goes through a series of trials and becomes extraordinary through them. It's a popular narrative that resonates across all humanity.

Heroes overcome *before* achieving their goals. It requires dedication and sacrifice. We're taught this from a very young age, although many of us missed the memo. Stories like *The Little Engine That Could* follow a blue locomotive as she pulls a train over a mountain. She repeats the phrase "I think I can! I think I can!" as she works, even though she isn't the fastest or most powerful train in the station. Similarly, *The Ugly Duckling* is a children's story about overcoming one rejection after another, until the duckling sees a swan and realizes where he belongs.

Now for a brief pop quiz—when the authors of these stories wrote them, what sounds more believable:

a. They wanted to make underdog choo-choo trains and ugly ducks feel better about themselves.

b. They used the trains and ducks as metaphors, or symbols of how human beings feel like underdogs or ugly/unwanted members of their community.

How many steam engines have you consoled for feeling down about themselves? How many ducks have waddled up to you for comfort because the other ducks think they're ugly? These are objects and animals! They don't care about being bigger, or more beautiful or handsome. They don't wrestle with body image or managing their emotions through eating. (I've never seen an obese duck, have you?) They just do what they're programmed to do. Only human beings despair and get discouraged about themselves.

One patient tucked his head in his hands and sobbed, sitting in the chair across from me. For months we had worked together, and he'd found success in small wins. But when things got hard, he fell off the wagon, and slipped back into old habits. His moment of weakness devastated him. In his mind, all the hard work he had put in counted for nothing—as if a slip back into old habits somehow "zeroed" everything he had achieved. In truth, he had simply stumbled. He was still headed in the right direction. Falling back into an old habit after making strides feels like self-betrayal—but it isn't. To this man, his mistake felt massive, but I knew from experience he could easily get back on track.

I reached across and put my hand on his shoulder and gave it a light squeeze. "Hey," I murmured, until he looked up at me. "What is your goal? I want you to remember it because this little storm, this hiccup, is not what we wanted or expected... but it's here. So let's come up with a plan for how to move forward." Eventually, he calmed down. Together, we came up with a plan to get him back on track.

Popular media portrays success as "simple," and, "overnight," a product of chance. This couldn't be further from the truth. Influencers who go viral, musicians who shoot to the top of the charts, or athletes who win championships go through a process before they achieve success. The process involves a lot of failure! They practice and cultivate their talent until it matures. One of my favorite sayings goes, "Amateurs practice until they can get something right; professionals practice until they can't get it wrong."

Your job, with each little step you take, is to become a *professional*—at drinking six cans of soda instead of eight, followed by two cans instead of six, followed by water instead of soda, and on down the line. Walk 500 feet, walk 1000 feet, walk one mile, walk three miles. Run 250 feet, run 700 feet, run 1500 feet, run one mile, run three miles. Anyone—and I mean *anyone*—can become professional with small steps like these.

"Small Steps" Are Lifelong

Though I'm in the best shape of my life, I recognize I'm not "done." I haven't stopped the practice of planning and executing small steps. I haven't hit a magic number that says I can stop everything and go back to my old habits. I have no plans to slow down or stop improving myself. One more time for the people in the back rows: *lifestyle, lifestyle, lifestyle.*

For me, small steps are a lifelong habit. Once I achieve a goal, I set a new one and develop a plan of action. Even as I write, I'm currently restarting Ironman training. Though I'm much healthier than I was when I trained for my first Ironman, I still have to acclimate my body for the race. Each day, I push myself to go on longer runs, swims and bike rides.

In truth, my bike is killing me. Riding for one hour is extremely taxing, because the familiarity isn't there. After my last Ironman, I stopped doing long bike rides because I focused on improving elsewhere. Now that I'm training for an Ironman again, I have to work back up to the ability to stay on a bike for 5-6 hours.

Even in good physical shape, this is difficult. I'm in a tucked-in position with elbows touching knees, hunched over, listening to the constant hum of the trainer (over and over and over). There's a computer that tells me my output, cadence, and heart rate. But as I stare at the screen for multiple hours, my body becomes tight. My back and neck cramp up and the tension builds across my shoulders.

I get used to it as I push on. But during the first several weeks of training, I want to raise my torso. The urge to slow down, stand and stretch is overwhelming. I must conquer my physical being and make my body become "one" with the bike. Distractions like TV shows help take my mind off it a little, but distraction isn't the point. The point of the exercise is to embrace discomfort and push myself through it. I'm doing this to develop high, consistent output and cadence, so I can do it for longer and longer without losing momentum.

I've accepted and embraced discomfort. That too requires small steps. With each ride, I hang on longer, and longer, until I can stay crouched in position for hours.

This also means going on longer bike rides, in terms of distance. My "small steps" there are related to performance. I tell myself, "I'm going to stay at a certain heart rate for ten minutes." Or I say, "My cadence is going to stay above 70 for the next five minutes." I view these goals as small challenges, opportunities to compete with myself and get better each time.

If I'm running for 20 minutes, I break those minutes into four clusters of five minutes each. As the clusters tick by I tell myself, "If I did that one, I can do another." I celebrate the win and that I'm able to continue the workout. I reaffirm myself when self-doubt creeps in and that voice in the back of my mind whispers, "This is too hard."

I also have small steps for the business side of life.

Currently I'm growing a new business, outside the world of healthcare. We're working in the real estate industry. To tell you the truth, I don't know much about this field yet. I often feel lost. I wonder if I've stepped into something completely over my head and that maybe I shouldn't have gone into real estate to begin with.

As these imposter thoughts creep in, I remember to break my real estate goals into small steps. With the pace of daily life, running the healthcare side of my business, training, and spending time with my family, I know I must start *very* small. My goals fit into a timeline that stretches over two years. At the end of those two years, I list the income I want to achieve because of those goals.

After doing this, tackling the unknown of the real estate market feels more manageable. I am making progress, and I feel less like an imposter. Today, I currently manage several different properties and understand the business better than I used to. I have a plan in place that requires me to devote a small amount of time to real estate each day. And like pieces in a puzzle, completing those steps leads to the finished product: a successful, profitable real estate business.

I give you these examples because I want "small steps" to help you on *more* than just your physical journey. Setting goals can help you get massive results *anywhere*. You can finally write your book, master an instrument, build a thriving business, or take the dream vacation you thought you couldn't afford. I want you to develop a lifelong habit of doing this, so you can get more out of life than you ever imagined!

How "Small Steps" Stack Up

Neglecting our physical health forces us to live in a false world, where negative emotions multiply. It's stressful, so we manage those uncomfortable feelings by turning to habits that make our problems worse. It's not a coincidence that the phrase "weight loss" includes a word associated with *losing*. The more weight you gain, the more you feel ... like a loser. It's too bad we can't say "weight winning," because *winning* is what truly leads to weight *loss*.

I love introducing the concept of small steps, and watching patients get their first "wins." Wins start a new trend where people break free of self-imposed limitations. The illusions people hold onto that "they can't do it," they're "permanently stuck" or "nothing works" begin to dissolve. They shed their "loser" mentality, and they begin to believe in themselves again.

As wins stack up, the mental shift arrives. People find the courage to take on greater challenges. By the way they talk and react, I can usually sense their shift from fixed to growth mindset. Despite the discomfort of their first small change, they realize—"I'm okay! I survived! That wasn't as terrible as I thought!" And success is as habit-forming as anything; once you've tasted it, you want more.

I love seeing emotions and countenances change. No more beaten-down faces, staring at the floor. It's as if someone placed rose-colored glasses on the crook of their nose; they're suddenly optimistic and confident. I see less hunching and drooping, fewer buried heads, and I hear subtle changes in their voices. They sit up straighter, their shoulders go back, their eyes twinkle, and they smile more. There's excitement about the opportunities ahead. They finally feel like they're in charge of the life they live.

Then come the physical changes: "My clothes fit better, my friends notice me, and they comment on how good I look." These moments are golden; we all do better with validation. We naturally stick close to people who appreciate us. Social and emotional approval from other human beings is very important. When the tribe validates your changes, it's next-level motivation.

Suddenly, people want to attend social events. They no longer feel the need to hide. Their "hermit" tendencies fade into the past. They stop "stepping away" when their friends want to take group photos. They become more outgoing and eager to join in, meet new people and experience new things. Their eyes open to new opportunities. They are more active and less passive about life in general.

Soon, others start asking the question—"What did you do? How do I do it too?" This is another golden mile marker on the journey. When you make progress, not only will you receive validation, but others will seek to learn how you did it and want it for themselves. Now, suddenly, *you're a leader*. That's a huge sign of progress. When people look to you for leadership and guidance, it encourages you to push further, and find out what other "walls" you've set up around yourself that need to be knocked down.

Do you understand now? Is it sinking in, just a little bit, that you don't have to leap over tall buildings with a single jump? You have the power to do the *tiniest* things ... and it's often the tiniest things that lead to avalanches. That's how I went from being on death's doorstep to running all these Ironmans. And you can have your own story of triumph, if you'll start small and lead yourself, gently but firmly, to becoming more today than you were yesterday.

Chapter 8:

BUILDING YOUR
SUPPORT NETWORK

When I was inspired to try new fad diets, I'd make the mistake of telling *everyone* about my plans. With each one I tried, I began full of confidence that I could make a real change this time. I would give it my all—for a few days—then inevitably fall back into my old habits.

Imagine how draining this was on my support network—my social circle.

Like the proverbial broken clock that's "right twice a day," I'd get excited about making a change. I'd set myself on a new path, with the promise of restoring my health. And everyone who loved and supported me would get excited *with* me. They would listen to my dreams, help me come up with a plan, and high five me the first time I did whatever the "fad" diet required. Then, it would get too hard, and I'd decide that it wasn't worth the discomfort. Inevitably, I'd quit.

I left my support system hanging, again and again. How many times did they have to push me to do something I didn't want to do for myself? After observing my pattern of giving up, why would they believe me if I came to them with yet *another* fad diet? It was like the parable of "The Boy Who Cried 'Wolf!'"

If you make big proclamations and fail to follow through on what you said you would do, eventually your supporters won't take you seriously. So be ready for it—if you've started and stopped a lot of programs, you may get a few raised eyebrows when you show your supporters this book and tell them what you plan to do. Some may even verbalize their doubts to your face. You can't let that get to you—this is new, and they can only go from your track record.

It's up to you to earn their trust and confidence again.

When Others Doubt You

When I started my journey, several naysayers and detractors stood in my way. At first, I was angry with them. How could they leave me out to dry when I was making progress towards big change? This time was different! But as I thought about it, I realized—they had good reason to doubt. I didn't keep the promises I'd made before. I had to accept the fact that their lack of support was largely my fault.

They'd learned their energy was wasted on encouragement because I didn't follow through. I needed to show them I was capable of change and that I did mean what I said. I told myself that no matter anyone's reaction, I would stick with this plan. I would regain the trust of my supporters.

Does any of this sound familiar? Have you ever alienated your support network? If so, as you start the process of small and meaningful change, you'll need to stick to your path for a while before they'll trust you again. I know the difficulty of this journey. Along the way, I experienced suspicion, envy, and derision. Usually, this would make me shut down and completely halt my progress. But this time was different.

Let's review each response that I got from people. Then we'll talk about how you work through them:

1. Suspicion

Along your journey, there will be people who completely dismiss your dreams and goals, simply because they have a fixed mindset. The last thing they'd believe is that anything is possible. Let's just call them "naysayers."

I believe many of us have naysayers in our social circles. Their dismissals might come coated in sugar: "You're fine just the way you are." Or they might be downright rude, "Do you think you can actually lose that much weight?" To them, the whole idea is absurd, like living in a fantasy world. They've closed their minds off, and they don't want to hear a different viewpoint.

I don't need to tell you—the old Casey would not have pushed through resistance like this. Unless you make the shifts we've already covered, you will find it difficult to overcome, too. People will hand you excuses to quit on a silver platter. Some of them will tell you straight up, even if they think they mean well. (Almost none of them do.)

2. Envy

Some people *sound* encouraging … but they carry hidden motives that undermine your progress.

One day, as I talked about running small distances, and going farther and farther each week, a friend shook his head and said, "You should be careful and slow down, you could hurt yourself. I tried that and it didn't end well."

Now, the old Casey would have heeded this warning. In fact, I would have likely used this statement as permission to quit. But the new Casey, the one with a growth mindset, recognized the comment for what it was: envy.

You see, some people don't want you to succeed, because it exposes their mediocrity. They project their failures onto you because failure is all they know. My friend's language implied that because he got hurt, I would too. And if I stopped, he wouldn't have to face the fact that I'd proved him wrong. But if I succeeded, what would that say about him?

Envy is sneaky. I don't know what exactly was in my friend's heart, but I knew that if I listened to it, I'd sabotage my own progress. You must learn to accept these comments for what they are, and don't let them deter you. The right people give you *constructive* criticism when necessary, and encouragement the rest of the time.

3. Derision

Others might try to convince you to train *harder* and *faster*. It's a veiled way of diminishing or badmouthing your progress.

Each person has a different health journey, but some people are convinced that what worked for them will work for everyone else. So, you might feel pressure to start where they started instead of where you are. For me, this looked like a fellow runner who said, "Why don't you just run a mile a day instead of 500 feet? It might be hard at first, but if you push through, you'll get it."

Once upon a time, I would have been embarrassed by his words. I would have wondered if I should listen to him. I might have accepted that I wasn't trying hard enough. Then I would likely feel depressed that I couldn't do things others seemed to do easily. This train of thought would have derailed my growth.

Your journey will look different from others. Some things are harder, and some are easier. I had to be realistic about what I could do at that point, and work to build capacity at my own pace. Otherwise, I'd have taken on more than I could handle. As author Jason Todd says, "Love *your* journey."

How to Succeed in Spite of Doubters

Suspicion, envy, and derision are real—but beatable. With each form of resistance, I've developed strategies to overcome them. I hope they will help you when you encounter resistance from others. They are:

1. **Center yourself**. Remember who you are. Remember where you are in your journey. And remember *why* you do what you do. You have a growth mindset now. You're a new person. Nobody can take your "why" away from you.

2. **Remember**: Just because someone suggests something, doesn't mean you have to act on it. Just because they excel in one area doesn't make them an expert in others. It's impossible for another person to walk in your shoes. They don't know everything in your past, which affects how you do things. Even if they sincerely want to help, you must take their encouragement with a grain of salt.

3. **Consider the source** or motive of the person speaking. Are they angry at themselves? Are they trying to escape from their own responsibilities? What pain do they have to make them act this way? Do you need to distance yourself from them? These answers will give you clarity into whether their words carry weight. If you don't trust someone to hold your money, don't give their comments about your journey too much thought.

4. **Be prepared** to verbally confront people. I've had several scenarios where I said, "I hear what you have to say, but I'm doing it anyway." This is your life, you're responsible for you, and no one else can dictate your actions. Do not let others live your life for you!

When people doubt me today, it still triggers me. I feel old Casey creeping in, asking, "Can I quit now?"

It's okay to go through this process. You're allowed to be sad when your social circle shows a lack of support. But you can't let them stop you. It's time to show them what you're really made of. After a few months, when my changes became real and people could see I wasn't going to give up, they began to encourage me and believe in what I said once more. I had regained their trust. I'd regained *my own* trust. It felt good.

I also proved some other people wrong … and that felt good too.

Company Makes a Difference

You will need to avoid certain people. It's a harsh reality of any self-improvement journey. As patients come in and out of my office, I'm always keen to see the people they talk about or bring along with them. Each client I've worked with is deeply influenced by the company they keep. As someone who helps them along the journey, I pay attention to their outside influences.

Losing weight resembles battling addiction. If you were addicted to drugs, and stepped into a Narcotics Anonymous meeting, a common discussion topic would be *who you spend your time with*. When people manage substance abuse, the importance of separating yourself from your former environment is a huge part of recovery. The company you keep *will* make or break your journey.

I'm not saying you should immediately cut off 20-year friendships. But during this change, you should focus on building lifelong relationships with people who encourage and hold you accountable. If you let others in your life halt your progress, you run the risk of returning to bad habits.

I once worked with a client who lost a significant amount of weight. They followed each step of the program, improved their diet, started exercising, and shifted their mentality. They felt better than they had in years! But they lacked community. They tried to recruit their friends into going to the gym and eating healthier together, but none of them were willing to make changes. As we sat in my office one day, I could tell this client felt bad. They picked at the arm of the chair across from me, and barely spoke. Eventually I asked, "Is anything bothering you right now?"

They sighed and nodded, "Not one of my friends has started to encourage me. I have made obvious physical changes, but none of them have commented on my progress. And *none* of them want to join me in trying to get healthy."

We talked about a few choices this client could make to engage other communities. There were places where they could find like-minded friends. But they weren't interested; they chose to stick with the same group of friends and keep trying to gain their support.

Ultimately, they settled for hanging out with the same group, in the same places, with the same habits, and stopped coming to the clinic altogether. It broke my heart to see it.

If you hang around people who discourage you, your difficulty level will go through the roof. Your social circle should eventually see your progress and *congratulate* you on it. If that doesn't happen, it's time to find a new circle—because without one, eventually the rock (you) will be worn down by the water (them).

Don't let this happen to you.

In my own journey, I had to intentionally reduce time with certain people. With a few of them, I had to cut ties completely. Today, I guard my time and exposure to certain people like a hawk. Why?

1. You are the sum of the five people you spend the most time with (thanks, Jim Rohn).
2. You are highly influenced by people around you, and you *will* pick up on their habits. So be careful who you spend your time with.

I'm so vigilant with who I allow in my life, that it's become a family joke: "I keep my scissors sharp." If people start to influence me in a negative way, I cut them off; they *have* to go.

Get around people who help you *grow*, full stop.

I like to look at it this way: Certain people have different levels of access to the areas in my house. They are:

- Bedroom people
- Living room people
- Front porch people
- Front yard people
- People on the other side of the fence

Bedroom people are the ones closest to you, who know you intimately. My bedroom people include my wife, my kids, very close friends and certain coaches and mentors who walked with me through my transformation. Living room people include friends and family who are supportive and encouraging, but not closely engaged. I enjoy interacting with front porch and yard people ... but only for short bursts. And the people on the other side of the fence? Yeah ... I don't do much beyond politely saying, "Hello."

Keep in mind—except for my wife and kids, none of these people are permanent residents in their locations. You can have your access revoked at any time, and the quickest way to do it is to be negative and destructive to me or my family.

Also understand this: when people change, *the nature of your relationship should change* too. I understand this can be painful if you were close, but you must do what's right for you. You deserve people in your life who build you up, and not the other way around. Keep your scissors sharp! If people hurt you, discourage you, or make you want to quit, then separate yourself.

The Ideal Support Network

What does the ideal support network look like? As I built mine, and helped others figure out theirs, I noticed a few things that make up an ideal support network. It should include champions, supporters, resistors, and bystanders.

Champions

Your ultimate champion should be like the "bedroom" person I defined above—constantly and closely supportive. Ideally, they're familiar with or experienced in the journey you're taking, and they are always encouraging, always believing, always trusting, and always cheering.

When I prepared to compete in my first Ironman, my daughter told everyone at her school. I worried I would let her and others down—but my wife was there as my champion. She listened to my worries and reassured me that I could in fact do something that seemed impossible. She never lost faith in me.

Supporters

Supporters are usually "ahead" of you—people who've traveled in your shoes that can help you stay focused. Coaches often fit this profile; they specifically help people like you and understand your struggles. They are deep wells of knowledge, resources, and relationships to assist you in your growth.

If you find a mentor or coach who specifically helps people like you, stick close to them. They are the closest thing you can get to a "shortcut." While training for my Ironman, I worked with a variety of coaches. They were *exactly* what I needed. I took their processes seriously, and followed each step they gave me. As a result, they could tell when I was overreacting to a strain, or if I was at risk of injuring myself. I trusted them when they said things like, "Just a little more, keep trying, keep going." I knew I could do it because *they* knew I could do it.

But there's more than one way to skin a cat; a person doesn't need to be a coach to be a supporter. You can also find supporters who are on your same journey—either further along, matching you step for step, or not quite as far as you. We've built online community groups at Restoration Health and Wellness that bring our patients together so they can form new connections. Quite often, the groups' veterans will befriend brand-new members, and walk them through their journey.

Resistors

Some resistance toward your journey is good and noble. After all, every hero needs a trial to overcome.

Everyone needs natural resistors. Their skepticism will surface when you share your plans and dreams. They might be some of the people we talked about earlier, whose trust you must earn back. Some coaches are healthy resistors, because they *always* want to see proof before they acknowledge your progress. I think of people like Jillian Michaels from the *Biggest Loser* reality TV series ... She was known for being hard-nosed and uncompromising, even as she got tremendous results for the contestants she trained.

Wherever loyal skepticism comes from, accept it for the challenge it is. Don't mistake someone who isn't "easily impressed" for a naysayer. At the right moment, "tough love" might be just what the doctor ordered.

Bystanders

A quick definition for bystanders—we're not talking about people you pass on the street who are unaware of your existence. A *bystander* is someone who knows (or knows of) you, and they're loosely aware of what you're going through.

Bystanders make themselves known in surprising moments. They are *always* watching, even if they don't admit it. They might be envious of/inspired by you and your journey. Sometimes they might comment on your photos, telling you how lucky you are to make such progress (when you and I know full well—it has nothing do with luck). Or you might get a message years later saying, "You really inspired me."

Every big change you make will include bystanders along the way. Acknowledge their presence, but don't work for them or their recognition. Work only for yourself and let them respond or react however they do.

Now, it's time to think about where the people in your immediate circle fall into these categories.

Cherish your champions and supporters. Think how much more motivated you feel in a conversation where you tell them about your wins. If you report something exciting in your life or a milestone you hit, do they light up with excitement and congratulate you? Do they ask you good questions and share in the joy with you? If so, they're the ones you hold closest; they're your bedroom people.

In the meantime, let your resistors and bystanders say what they say, while you weigh their comments carefully. Don't rush to misinterpret their skepticism or feedback as negative, but make a note of it, and discuss it among your champions and supporters. Sometimes, especially with resistors, they'll notice something you're neglecting, and emphasize it. That's valuable information to know if everyone else has somehow missed it! And if bystanders gravitate toward you because you're inspiring them, you know—you're transcending your former life, and becoming a true leader. Leadership begins with leading *yourself*, and it's only when you are in full control of yourself that you can command respect from others.

The Support System "Click"

Have you ever had the opportunity to hang out with a group of people who just "get" you? Almost from the start, they know what you're going through, how you feel and what you need.

They could be old friends or new friends, family, or spouses—but they have your best interests at heart and enjoy your company. Think about what this does for you mentally. We crave validation and acceptance from others. All our silly social norms and odd habits stem from this need—to be accepted by our fellow human beings.

So, what happens to your mindset if you find that group? I'll give you the answer: You start to run like a well-oiled machine.

When my support system began to click, I found the daily encouragement, stability, consistency, and accountability I needed. The further I went, the more automatic it became. In the darker years before my transformation, I might have gone for months or *years* before encountering the feeling of being among the right group of people. But the more I worked to become the man I am today, the less I had to work at finding support and encouragement. When you're working hard to be a better version of you, people come out of the woodwork to reinforce your mission.

I've seen the same thing happen for the patients at our clinics. The more they focus on developing a strong support network, the more they overcome resistance. They feel more positive about problems they face and eagerly hold themselves accountable. Their success attracts others without effort, and they find everything they need to charge toward the finish line.

I can remember crossing a few finish lines on my own, without my support network. Even though it was still a success, it somehow felt "less successful" when there was no one to celebrate with. In those races, I would count the telephone poles that went by, just to stay motivated. I would say to myself, "You can do one more telephone pole." But the races where someone stood at the finish line, waiting for me? Well, I no longer had to count telephone poles. I was *going* to get there.

As the old African proverb says, "If you want to go fast, go by yourself. If you want to go far, go with a team." We're not supposed to be on mountaintops every single day. As individuals, we will fail. Success is not constant, no matter who you have in your corner. You will experience hills and valleys in your journey. But valleys can be extraordinarily beautiful, especially if you have someone to share them with.

Some of the greatest treasures I've collected from my journey are the memories I share with my champions—*about the way things used to be*. Sometimes, they come across a photo of me in my old days, and they remark, "I look back and I can't believe that was you. It seems like ancient history."

Me too. I can't believe it was me, either.

No matter who you are or how good you are, you need allies to help you think. Another set of eyes allows you to see past your biases to a clearer understanding of the truth. We weren't created to be by ourselves. Back in Eden, man was created for relationships with God and with other people. According to my mentor Aaron Walker, author of *View From The Top*, "Isolation is the enemy of excellence."

We can't be the whole puzzle. We're just one piece of it. At the same time, the beauty of the full picture isn't complete without us. When you pick your team, you can either enlist them silently, or approach them and state your intentions out loud. I alternate, depending on the situation; I am vocal with some while silent with others. I'm watching and learning from them.

Whether they know it or not, they are a part of my support network, because they inspire me.

Picking the right team bleeds into my clinical work as well.

At Restoration Health and Wellness, some employees have been on staff ten to twelve years, while others have barely been on the job for three weeks. But I know I couldn't do five percent of what I do right now without them. When I had limited staff, I had to stop seeing patients because I didn't have enough time in the day to handle the load. Thank God, that's no longer a problem. Together, we help more people today than we ever have.

So, who belongs in *your* support system? Are there people you need to ask for help? Are there others you need to cut out? Now that you understand the different roles in a support network, and how much they influence you—how can you adjust your circle for the best results? Don't do this alone; do yourself a favor and find the people who inspire you.

CONCLUSION

As we close, I urge you to think deeply about this question:

Are you happy with your current situation?

Stop. Pause. Read the question again. Take time to come up with a real answer.

Are you where you want to be with your health, mindset, career, and relationships? My guess, because you picked up this book, is, "No." And if you're like me, you're frustrated. You've tried everything and got nowhere. I see this cycle again and again when patients walk through the door of my clinic. It's disheartening and demotivating for them because they're stuck.

But for you, today can be different. Today could be the day you change everything.

I wrote this book to help you get your life back— the life you were really meant to live. A life you can be proud of. You took the first step by seeking help. When you picked up this book, you were searching for a new path. Congratulations! Many people pass up the opportunity and remain stuck in their ways. They want to change, but they don't know how to do it. You took action by reading this book.

And now, you have the tools to make small consistent changes that lead to huge ones. Whether you have 50 or 150 lbs to lose, you're prepared. You know the stakes; the journey will be filled with discomfort, doubt, anger, guilt, and fear. But you also know these temporary challenges are worth the discomfort. A new you awaits on the other side of this journey. Your future self will thank you for every change you make.

Together, we've reviewed eight key concepts:

- **Gratitude** comes first; we can't make physical changes without changing how we think.
- We can't expect to grow if we reject **possibility**; we must believe anything is possible.
- **Difficulty** is next; we must have faith that we can do hard things.
- Today is not yesterday; we can become **better today than we were yesterday**.
- **Discomfort** is part of the deal; learn to be comfortable in uncomfortable situations.

- More than losing body weight, we're transforming from a **fixed to growth mindset**.
- Slow and steady wins the race, and we achieve daily wins through **small steps**.
- We rise and fall on the company we keep, so we must build a solid **support network**.

I want you to remember: Change is within your reach.

No matter your situation, if you follow the steps in this book, you can make progress. I encourage you to record the changes as they happen, just as I did within my race journal entries. It might be the biggest change you make in your life, and I promise you will want to look back at your progress. And when things are difficult, reviewing your progress will offer extra motivation.

If you need help, I invite you to reach out and connect. You can find me on my Instagram @imlivinoutloud, or you can contact us directly on my clinic's website at restorationhealthwellness.com.

If I can do it, so can you. Start changing everything today!

Casey Elkins

ABOUT THE AUTHOR

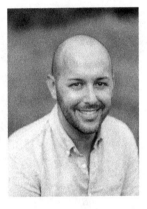

Casey Elkins is a husband, father, business owner, college professor, and IRONMAN World Championship competitor.

After a near death experience, Casey transformed his life and lost nearly 100 pounds, on his way to competing in over a dozen IRONMAN Triathlons.

The founder and owner of Restoration Health and Wellness in Mobile, Alabama, Casey has a doctorate degree in nursing, two master's degrees and devotes his professional life to inspiring others to implement healthy lifestyle changes.

In addition to his IRONMAN performances, Casey has completed numerous marathons and other endurance sports events.

A free ebook edition is available with the purchase of this book.

To claim your free ebook edition:

1. Visit MorganJamesBOGO.com
2. Sign your name CLEARLY in the space
3. Complete the form and submit a photo of the entire copyright page
4. You or your friend can download the ebook to your preferred device

Morgan James
BOGO™

A **FREE** ebook edition is available for you
or a friend with the purchase of this print book.

CLEARLY SIGN YOUR NAME ABOVE

Instructions to claim your free ebook edition:
1. Visit MorganJamesBOGO.com
2. Sign your name CLEARLY in the space above
3. Complete the form and submit a photo
   of this entire page
4. You or your friend can download the ebook
   to your preferred device

Print & Digital Together Forever.

Snap a photo

Free ebook

Read anywhere

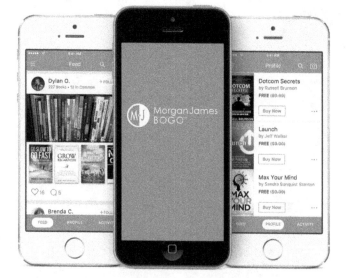